Art Therapy and Psychology

Taking an interdisciplinary approach, Robert Gray offers a thorough and well-rounded clinical guide to exploring the depth of the unconscious through art in psychotherapy. He emphasises the clinical relevance of art therapy and critically highlights ideas around evidence-based practice and the link to cognitive behavioural therapy. Gray suggests specific ways of engaging with clients and their images, such as uncovering life scripts, changing neural pathways through Creative Mind Ordering, and addressing traumatic experiences through the Jungian Self-Box. He shows how artists and psychotherapists can make a transformational difference by combining 'art as therapy' and 'art in therapy' with a scientific approach and a spiritual awareness. He argues a clear framework that bridges the unmeasurable and spontaneous part of psychotherapy through art, along with the work with the unconscious and the clarity of a scientific method, can help facilitate long term change.

Art Therapy and Psychology is hands-on and rich with supportive study tools and numerous case studies with which the reader can relate. This book is essential reading for art therapists in training and in practice, psychologists and mental health professionals looking to establish or grow their expertise.

Robert P. Gray is an art therapy lecturer from Germany, with degrees in art therapy, psychology and theology. He is Director of the College for Educational and Clinical Art Therapy, Australia. As an Australian psychologist, he leads the field in art therapy with his unique integration of psychological techniques and spiritual practices.

"This book is for art therapists and mental health professionals who would like to expand their repertoire of art interventions to connect with and aid in the healing process of individuals with various challenges. Like the title suggests, numerous art therapy exercises are delineated which explore Gray's ideas through in-depth case studies, including verbal exchanges between patient and therapist. Gray goes beyond a set of interventions and explores various theories that inform his practice: psychoanalysis, positive psychology, neurobiological science, and evidence-based theories such as CBT. This practice-oriented book is a constructive addition to the art therapist's tool box."

Marcia L. Rosal, PhD, ATR-BC, HLM.
Professor Emerita, Florida State University, USA

Art Therapy and Psychology

Psychology

A Step-by-Step Guide for Practitioners

Robert P. Gray

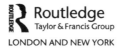

Routledge
Taylor & Francis Group

LONDON AND NEW YORK

First published 2019
by Routledge
2 Park Square, Milton Park, Abingdon, Oxon OX14 4RN

and by Routledge
52 Vanderbilt Avenue, New York, NY 10017

Routledge is an imprint of the Taylor & Francis Group, an informa business

British Library Cataloguing-in-Publication Data
A catalogue record for this book is available from the British Library

Library of Congress Cataloging-in-Publication Data
A catalog record for this book has been requested

ISBN: 978-0-8153-5590-8 (hbk)
ISBN: 978-0-8153-5591-5 (pbk)
ISBN: 978-1-351-12905-3 (ebk)

Typeset in Minion
by Apex CoVantage, LLC

Dedicated to Jembe and India. To inspire them.

Contents

Introduction   1

1 Foundations   6

2 Positive art therapy   17

3 Representational images, projective drawings and
   the House-Tree-Person (HTP) task   30

4 Life Script: Create an alternative script   43

5 Goals: Overcome obstacles   56

6 Abstract art and the self-picture mind map   67

7 Self-Box: Become authentic and integrate traumatic memories   80

8 Creative Mind Ordering (CMO): Change neural pathways   93

9 Advancing art therapy and cognitive behaviour therapy (CBT)   112

10 Group art therapy   127

   Pseudonyms   138
   Acknowledgments   139
   Index   140

Introduction

Art therapy is often imagined as a kind of creative playground. The therapist supervises a process that is quite therapeutic in its own way, but it often has little bearing on concrete outcomes. Art therapy however, can be much more than that. It can alter core beliefs or schemas that often underpin lifelong troublesome ways of being in the world. Art therapy, as I will explain throughout this book and through each art therapy exercise, can be the key to unlocking the door of the unconscious, and allowing for an in depth healing process to begin.

If you've ever marvelled at the primitive sketches of the Lascaux caves or the rock markings of Arnhem Land in Australia, you've witnessed the power of imagery. Imagery has been used to create and share narratives since the earliest recordings of time. In fact, long before modern language, movable type and social media, images, symbols and objects were used to communicate deep cultural and personal meanings. It's no surprise that death and loss features heavily in ancient imagery, since imagery has the power to both define what it is to be human and to elucidate and transform difficult human experience. From masks worn for self-preservation and protection to the use of symbols to heal sickness, art is a seasoned healer that transcends time and verbal language. The well-known and respected American art therapist Judith Rubin (1978, p. 206) said, "from the cave to the Sunday painter, normal people in ordinary settings have been using art for personally helpful purposes". Our theoretical understanding of how imagery works and how art can heal is a mystery to some extent; however, a great deal of study and development of the psychological effects of imagery has taken place in the last hundred years to bring art therapy into the forefront as a major contributor of the healing practices.

When art therapy was in its infancy, around the time of Adrian Hill, who first began using art therapy with hospital patients, psychoanalysis and analytical psychology were enjoying a kind of heyday. The famous Sigmund Freud and his equally famous student Carl Gustav Jung gained celebrity status, paving the way for talk-based counselling methodologies. They theorised that images in the form of dreams were like an access code to the unconscious.

Although imagery played a major role, representations in drawings or paintings were, funnily enough not considered.

> We experience it [a dream] predominantly in visual images . . . Part of the difficulty of giving an account of dreams is due to our having to translate these images into words. "I could draw it," a dreamer often says to us, "but I don't know how to say it."
>
> (Freud, 1916–1917, p. 90)

Freud's great frustration might have been one of the contributing factors in the development of art therapy. Consequently, this quote can be found in many art therapy books. Words are our main form of communication, but some ideas are difficult, or impossible to articulate. Images represent an alternative medium for expression and communication. Once experiences are externalised in images however, novel words often start emerging by seeing the artwork or reflecting on the art making process.

Whether you're a psychologist, a social worker, a counsellor working in mental health, family therapy, or an artist wishing to channel your passion into helping others, the knowledge you will acquire from reading this book will equip you to co-pilot journeys to parts of clients' selves crucial to healing. You will help them to live the life they couldn't otherwise imagine while gaining deep personal insight, yourself. Of course, reading a book does not make you an art therapist. There is much more to learn than can be done by enrolling into a course with experts in the field at a university or a college, however this book will make a huge difference by giving you additional information and knowledge that you might not find anywhere else. By using image-making to access unconscious parts of the mind, you will, at the end of this book, be prepared to guide clients skilfully on their journey to uncharted, exciting parts of themselves. You will learn to collaborate with clients to make their unconscious conscious and help them realise the capacity to process and integrate what they didn't know was holding them back.

Unlike many verbal therapies, the therapeutic processes developed and detailed in these chapters, appoints the client as the expert and empowers them to find their own solutions by interpreting their guided image-making. As you can imagine, it can be immensely empowering to a client when they find their own answers within.

The recent revival in Australia towards 'health and art' groups indicates an increased interest in combination therapies using creative practice and talk therapy alongside medication. The techniques you will learn fuse evidence-based psychotherapeutic principles with verified neurobiological frameworks to both bypass and leverage language centres to unlock, process and transform. Imagine an elevator in a high-rise apartment building that only goes to certain floors unless you have a key tag. You will learn to give clients their own all-floors pass. As a fringe benefit, as you study, you will also undertake your own personal journey of discovery.

Although many theoretical models in psychotherapy have been applied to 'art as therapy' with the main focus on the process, and 'art in therapy'/art psychotherapy, focusing on the deeper meaning of the artwork, only a few have been adequately reflected in the literature and serve as models of intervention today

(Malchiodi, 2012). In my experience, the majority of art therapists view themselves as eclectic and use more than one of type of intervention. Ideally, however, an eclectic form of intervention does not mean choosing random approaches from various backgrounds; it means choosing approaches carefully according to the individual client, the presenting problem and the situational variables. Also art therapists, like psychologists (Prochaska & Norcross, 2013), need a commitment to an exact process of therapy, so we don't work with incompatible assumptions in a chaotic and possibly hazardous way. This book aims to help you find the right approach for your client and to commit yourself to a certain but flexible process of change. I like to borrow Wadeson's (2016) idea of essentially becoming 'selective eclectic'.

My work bridges art and psychology in a psychodynamic way. It expands on the medical behavioural model and the part of psychotherapy that can't be controlled, measured and instrumentalised. There is great danger in a medical model of art therapy that focuses only on symptoms and short-term practical solutions, very similar to a behaviour therapy approach that assumes the client is a blank slate where we can imprint new behaviours. I believe the medical model does not take adequate account of the complexity and uniqueness of our clients issues. Alternatively, many art therapy books that mainly focus on art as therapy, neglect the complexity of psychotherapy. There is a mystical belief inherent that art will do the job whether we understand the processes or not. Art as therapy might make a client feel better, but unfortunately, for someone with a serious issue who is coming to therapy for help, this is often not good enough. A clear approach and framework of art in therapy in facilitating change is required, which is what this book offers.

As a practising psychotherapist with more than 25 years' experience working with families and serious mental health disorders, I believe that the curative potential of 'pure' cognitive behavioural therapy (CBT), coined in the 1960s and 70s and recognised as the dominant psychotherapeutic paradigm, is limited. While it may eventually access unconscious thoughts underlying unhelpful behaviours and emotions, that level of depth may take years, which contradicts health insurance provisions for a limited number of subsidised sessions per year. It often then becomes a panacea, failing to provide lasting change, with adverse implications for both clients and society.

More and more psychologists are looking for something else to add to their expertise and talking therapies are not always sufficient on their own. Art therapists, on the other hand, have creative techniques as their strategy, but they are sometimes missing the understandings from psychological knowledge. If we take different therapeutic frameworks including behavioural science seriously, art therapists who only use art as therapy, have to consider some changes to their practice. Most art therapists might feel a bit uncomfortable with simplistic CBT and the medical model of quick solutions that aims at reducing symptoms. However, art therapists can learn a great deal from CBT evidence-based practice and similar approaches. We need not follow a rigid and narrow approach in psychotherapy. We should use our intuition and flexibility and not be constrained by fear of law suits. Nevertheless, CBT has taught me that sometimes we can be practical and that it is not always bad to be directive with clients. We are allowed to follow an agenda, and often can achieve amazing outcomes in this way. Also, while art therapy is founded on psychoanalytic and psychodynamic techniques, art therapists would be better off to integrate CBT and its useful elements, as well as other approaches, into their practice on an as-needs basis. For instance, once art therapy has fostered the client's insight into deep psychological problems, CBT may provide a method to rebuild thinking and behaviour.

Short-term therapy has become the norm and it challenges us to re-think what we do as art therapists. In our current environment, where the government and medical centres only support 5–10, sometimes 20 sessions, this presents a great challenge. CBT therapists struggle as well, but at least their approach allows them to be somewhat effective in the short term.

While I do believe as therapists we need to stand together, become politically active and demand more time for our clients with high needs, we also have to use therapies that work well within our time constraints. For this reason, in this book I have showcased, an approach of 'art as therapy' and especially 'art in therapy' with expeditious outcomes for short- and middle-term cases, where unconscious material can become conscious by simply looking at the artwork and facilitating a clear process, and where the client can discover their own answers.

On a practical note, please read the book from start to finish and resist the temptation to skip chapters, as there are many sequential ideas, just like an engaging story with a beginning, middle and end. This book is full of techniques, instructions and clear descriptions of how art therapy can be effective with clients, step by step. If certain techniques in this book appear too cognitive or too challenging for you or your young client or for the client who has a mental disability, you can simplify the techniques to make them fit. Art therapy approaches have to be as organic as our clients. It is much easier to simplify an approach than to make something basic, like colouring in, more interesting and insightful.

This book is also about the magic of the unknown. We need to follow our own intuition in the knowledge that we can't control everything in our lives. We have to leave some things unanswered. I feel that the artists among the readers are sure to feel at home with the art techniques. I hope that critical art therapists and opponents of the medical model, as well as clinical psychologists who follow evidence-based practice, are going to enjoy the book and find the different approaches as rewarding and beneficial as I have. My hope is that this work provides for positive outcomes for both you and your clients.

Robert Gray

Literature

Case, C., & Dalley, T. (2014). *The handbook of art therapy* (3rd ed.). London, New York: Routledge-Taylor & Francis Group.

Edwards, D. (2004). *Art therapy*. London: Sage.

Freud, S. (1916–1917). *Introductory letters on psychoanalysis* (Vol. 10). London: Hogarth Press.

Hill, A. (1948). *Art versus illness*. London: Allen & Unwin.

Kramer, E. (1971). *Art as therapy with children*. New York: Schocken Books-Chicago.

Malchiodi, C.A. (2012). Clinical approaches to art therapy. In C.A. Malchiodi (Ed.), *Handbook of art therapy* (pp. 53–140). New York: Guilford Press.

Naumburg, M. (1950). *Introduction to art therapy: Studies of the 'free' art expression of behaviour problem children and adolescents as a means of diagnosis and therapy*. New York: Teachers College Press.

Naumburg, M. (1953). *Psychoneurotic art: Its function in psychotherapy*. New York: Grune and Stratton.

Prochaska, J.O., & Norcross, J.C. (2013). *Systems of psychotherapy: A transtheoretical analysis* (8th ed.). Stamford: Cengage Learning.

Rubin, J.A. (1978). *Child art therapy*. New York: Litton Educational.

Rubin, J.A. (2016). Introduction. In Rubin, J.A. (Ed.), *Approaches to art therapy: Theory and technique* (pp. 1–14) (3rd ed.). New York, Oxon: Routledge.

Rubin, J.A. (2016). Discovery and insight in art therapy. In Rubin, J.A. (Ed.), *Approaches to art therapy: Theory and technique* (pp. 71–86) (3rd ed.). New York, Oxon: Routledge.

Ulman, E., & Dachinger, P. (1975). *Art therapy in theory and practice*. New York: Schocken Books-Chicago.

Wadeson, H. (2016). An eclectic approach to art therapy. In Rubin, J.A. (Ed.), *Approaches to art therapy: Theory and technique* (pp. 71–86) (3rd ed.). New York and Oxon: Routledge-Taylor & Francis Group.

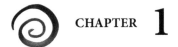

CHAPTER 1

Foundations

This book and you

A major part of this book is about you, about understanding yourself, and reflecting on the deeper meaning of your drawings, paintings and artworks that you are asked to produce from the methods described in the following pages. In my opinion, doing art within a specific framework is the best way for you to learn art therapy, so I have compiled my most tried and true methods, which I have used with clients for many years and which have worked successfully time and time again. You don't need to be an artist to do this. The methods and techniques are designed to help you observe your thoughts and emotions as you draw or paint and to be non-judgmental of the process. As you progress through the book you will find it easier to 'make space'. This means being in the moment and allowing things to happen and yourself to change. The methods help you to be more mindful or 'awareful' with all your thoughts, emotions, senses, body and spirit. At times you will notice if you are upset or angry as you draw, at other times you might find your spiritual side emerging, giving you greater insight into how you truly feel, as you uncover deeper levels of yourself in the artwork.

Art therapy helps us to explore who we are. There will be many instances when you will just *notice* what happens with your thoughts and feelings. Be aware and take notes when this happens, allow it to happen and reflect on it later. You might even choose to buy a personal journal to accompany the reading of this book. If a picture surprises you, irritates you or makes you upset, you have something to work with. This is a gift, a moment in time where your life can change for the better. You might want to talk to somebody about it, a friend, a partner or see an art therapist to help you with some of the issues that may come up for you.

In the process of art making one becomes engaged in the practice in such a way that observation skills become heightened. Each technique in the following chapters will involve you in this way, and as you take small steps into the journey of self-understanding, you will notice changes occurring on a deeper level, giving you greater insight, helping you be in the moment, as well as allowing you to be more perceptive of the life you want to lead, and more astute about the future you want to create.

Working with the unconscious mind

Freud's iceberg in art therapy

The development of art therapy and its profound usefulness as a healing practice can be historically linked to Sigmund Freud, the founder of psychoanalysis. Even though Freud has been criticised for many of his assumptions and theories, especially about sexuality, he contributed significantly to a field of knowledge that unleashed groundbreaking insights into human behaviour during a very restrictive period in history. His lack of understanding of women, and his theories on castration anxiety, penis envy, hysteria and many other assumptions have been highly debated. Many of Freuds contemporaries were women, who built on or criticised his work, and this interest created a snowball effect of advancements in neurology and psychotherapy around the world. Two pioneers in the field of art therapy, and whose work is intrinsically linked to Freud, are Margaret Naumburg and Edith Kramer. Both used Freud's understanding of the unconscious in their therapeutic art practice with patients (Tobin, 2015).

Even though Freud himself never used the image of an iceberg, it can be an extremely useful metaphor to help us understand the way he perceived and understood the relationship between our conscious and unconscious mind. The tip of the iceberg, above the water, represents the conscious mind while the bulk of mental content, in the unconscious, lies below the surface. What makes mental health issues so challenging is that, often, the content that prohibits optimal functioning is literally 'out of sight, out of mind' and liable to intrude upon consciousness without warning; without awareness of the culpable thoughts or beliefs. This is still valid 80 years after Freud. Have you ever wondered why you sometimes attract the same types of toxic people or run late for everything? Complicating matters further, the unconscious plays by different rules to those we assume to be true in conscious life. For instance, in the unconscious there is no time, which is why trauma can resurface as a relentless memory. In the presence of a trigger, the brain responds as though it *is* happening now – not 10 or 30 years ago. Since the unconscious mind is believed to be the 'driver' of what we really think, feel and do, this susceptibility means that gains made using talk-based methodologies in the here and now are often limited.

Take the dominant psychotherapeutic framework, cognitive behaviour therapy (CBT). The focus of CBT is on observable behaviour and conscious cognitions/ thoughts. Treatment focuses on changing dysfunctional assumptions, expectations and interpretations of events as well as negative self-talk into positive, healthy thinking (Hofmann, 2012). In the iceberg context, it works only at the 'tip', with thoughts and behaviours that can be consciously accessed.

Example: Client with the belief "I'm not a good mother."

Parent programs that use CBT may install an opposing, more adaptive or helpful thought ("I'm a good mother"), but might fail to address the underlying childhood issues and related beliefs that lie in her unconscious. If her worldview is built upon the experience of being told that she was no good at anything by a critical parent in her early childhood, her belief that she is a good mother will at best be superficial, fragile and susceptible to rupture with any suggestion that favours her not-good-enough belief.

Freud, Jung and others have observed and written, that imagery can be used to encourage a person's unconscious to rise into their consciousness. In psychoanalysis, the unconscious is described as "the part of the mind which you are not aware of but which affects behaviour and emotions" (Waite & Hawker, 2009, p. 762). Art can often bypass vulnerability and defence mechanisms inherent to verbal communication, making visible an image in one's inner world (Swan-Foster, 2016). By making the unconscious conscious, art therapy can enable fundamental 'shifts' that, in turn, alter conscious thoughts, feelings and behaviours for the better.

Emotions and the unconscious

Most practitioners have a basic understanding of how emotions affect the brain, a person's ability and function. Emotions like anger and grief, can play havoc with our lives, and can be detrimental to our well-being. Many of us are aware of how emotions that overwhelm us can cause us to lose focus on what we are doing. We may be unable to think of others, but only of ourselves, or on the emotion that is taking charge. Not being able to process highly charged emotions in ourselves can lead to long-term problems, even depression and anxiety. Frequently, traumatic experiences from early childhood are triggers for things we feel in our adult life. Even with the best of parenting and support we can still suffer intensely from an early age, which, in turn, will create many different negative feelings around grief and loss. These stored emotions, experiences or trauma stay in the body and in the unconscious, and, if unreleased, can make a person either overwhelmed with emotion, angry or numb, or any number of residual feelings can occur. This is often why depressed clients don't know why they are depressed. Depression can have a history of buried emotions. A great deal has been written about the need for talking about one's emotions in order to heal, however sometimes clients, especially depressed clients, aren't able to target what is causing them distress. It can be confusing, so they aren't able to discuss their deep feelings or problems, as they are not even consciously aware of them.

Art therapy works to uncover unconscious feelings, grief and trauma, 'stuck feelings' in the body and mind. I find it helps clients to access the hidden aspects of themselves, allowing them to understand their emotional condition. Art therapy can give a release to their experience, by allowing the emotion to surface, be acknowledged and be re-integrated. Once the unconscious becomes conscious and the deep-seated feelings become unstuck, a client is much more capable of talking about their problems, feelings and thoughts. So it is helpful to use a combination of art therapy for the unconscious work, together with a talking therapy like CBT, for consciously understanding ourselves.

Cognitive behaviour therapy (CBT) and psychoanalysis

The difference between the two

> The intellectual forebears of cognitive-behavioural therapies are found in the empirical-positivist tradition of American academic psychology rather than in the European philosophical attitudes that influenced Freud and many other psychodynamic therapists.
>
> (McWilliams, 2011)

Cognitive behavioural therapy, developed from cognitive therapy by the American psychologist Albert Ellis and psychiatrist Aaron Beck, and behavioural therapy (developed mainly by American academics including Watson, Wolpe, Meichenbaum, Skinner and Bandura to name a few), has similar goals to psychoanalysis. This approach can help clients overcome difficulties, change their behaviour, and move forward in their lives. Many of the CBT treatments have clearly demonstrated their effectiveness in reducing symptoms; however, these are best suited to clients who are in need of short-term therapy, 15 to 20 weeks. CBT is best suited for clients whose problems stem from more immediate issues, and where inaccurate thinking can be changed or modified in order to affect behaviour. McWilliams (2011) contended that some clients also prefer a more focused and directed treatment, complete with homework assignments.

Psychoanalysis and psychodynamic therapies are more contemplative processes that can take many years; the goal is to uncover the underlying unconscious schemata. Unlike CBT, it involves an emphasis on childhood and past experiences, on exploration of the unconscious, and on wishes, dreams, and fantasies (McWilliams, 2011).

CBT is similar to psychoanalysis in that there is an exploration of patterns in the patient's actions, thoughts, feelings, experiences and relationships (object relations). However, psychodynamic therapies differ in that they focus more on expression of emotion and the role of emotion in the client's life. The patient's efforts to avoid certain topics (i.e. resistance) is also examined, as the fear of change is often a strong unconscious motive. In psychoanalysis there is also an emphasis on the therapeutic relationship (transference and working alliance) (McWilliams, 2011).

Moreover, many with a psychodynamic sensibility could not work within a manualised CBT framework; it is too left-brained for many therapists and clients (McWilliams, 2011). There is often a need to help the client achieve balance in their life through therapy. Where clients might be too logical, too linear or unable to be spontaneous, it is important to stimulate right-brain thinking, whereby clients can be more open emotionally, less linear, and more wholistic (Carnevale, 2015).

On a final note: What I personally love about working with images and the unconscious is that "accidents can happen", as Case and Dalley (2014, p. 114) put it so discerningly. Working with a CBT approach can quickly achieve a directed and practical outcome. A great adjunct to art therapy. Within an art therapy approach however, you want to allow for 'accidents', chaos, confusion and contradictions.

Often, it is exactly these moments when 'accidents' happen that can be eye-opening for our clients. When something totally unexpected comes up this can make a huge difference.

In the following chapters we will examine how both approaches, and a variety of others, can coexist harmoniously for better client outcomes.

Exploring the official timeline of art therapy and psychology

- Early 1900s: Freud and Jung lead the way with the 'power' of the unconscious.
- 1930s: 'Art as therapy' is used in mental health institutions.
- 1940s: 'Art in therapy' (some authors call it 'art psychotherapy') began when psychiatrists, psychologists and art therapists started using drawings and paintings as a way to replace verbal communication, to prompt discussion, explore transference (of feelings from client to analyst), and countertransference (from analyst to client), and to tap into the unconscious material of their clients.
- 1950s: Behavioural therapy developed in opposition to psychoanalysis and the work with the unconscious. After the horrors of World War II, psychoanalysis, with its strong focus on the life instinct, which includes sexual instincts 'Eros', and the death instinct, destruction and death wish 'Thanatos' as core impulses, lost popularity, possibly out of a need for something more tangible, dependable, measurable and reliable. This was a crucial moment in history, where many psychologists moved away from working with the unconscious and art therapy. I believe the world was traumatised by this event and when people are affected by trauma, they like to be pragmatic and rational. They don't want to delve too deeply. Even if they reflect on the past, they want to focus on practical solutions in the present and concentrate on the future.
- 1960s: Cognitive therapy has been developed to deal with the shortcomings of behaviour therapy. It helped to identify thinking and how it affected us, i.e. sometimes people tend to do the right thing, but their thinking is not in it, which can cause them stress etc. You might be nice to your boss, but think otherwise and grumble.
- 1960s: Humanistic therapy is a third force (Maslow, 1968; Moon, 2016), opposing the determinism of dehumanising psychoanalysis and behaviour therapy. There is a strong belief that we are capable of healing ourselves, and the role of the therapist is 'just' to enable that. I personally see this approach as the baseline for all good therapy. We start here and then use different approaches in a decisive way. Consequently, we don't need to have all the answers and can be respectful and supportive towards the inner wisdom of our clients.
- 1970s: Behaviour therapy and cognitive therapy got 'married' and formed a powerful union, a paradigm of evidence-based practice for decades to come, continuing up to today.
- Today: Throughout all those years, art therapy has not disappeared, but has become more widely accepted and many psychologists who struggle with using CBT alone show an increased interest in working 'again' with the unconscious including art therapy.

Two types of art therapy

Of course, we can theoretically divide art therapy in many different ways, but over the last few decades this model has worked well for me, in a very practical way.

Despite its informal longevity, reaching back to the primitive cave paintings, art therapy only really emerged as a therapeutic paradigm in the 1930s and 1940s. A British artist, educator and the author of *Art Versus Illness*, Adrian Hill appears to be the first person who used the term '*art therapy*' to link art making to the therapeutic process (Edwards, 2004). Hill (1948) believed that the practice of art could turn society away from war, by encouraging appreciation of artistic creativity. Around the same time, Edith Kramer (1971) introduced the idea of '*art as therapy*', eschewing verbal interpretation in psychoanalysis for the therapeutic scope of the creative process.

In sync with the psychoanalytic practice of her days, and different to Kramer's focus on the art as therapy process, Margaret Naumburg's art psychotherapy had a strong focus on '*art in therapy*'/*art psychotherapy*, where unconscious material was uncovered through the analysis of the artwork (Ulman & Dachinger, 1975). She believed that the drawn images represent inner images of the client and can facilitate and lead into discourse or substitute it while being in therapy (Naumburg, 1953). These two cornerstones of art therapy have prevailed until today.

There are art therapists today like Cathy Malchiodi (2012) who witnessed the aftermath of September 11 in the US, and highly recommend an art as therapy approach in trauma work. Others like Caroline Case and Tessa Dalley (2014) from the UK, also acknowledged the importance of the psychoanalytic approach in art therapy, allowing inner experiences from the unconscious to become conscious and verbal. Their special interest being the therapeutic relationship. *Note: Psychologists among my readers, this should not be mistaken for Carl Rogers' (1951) humanistic and client-centred approach that facilitates a strong therapeutic relationship through interpersonal warmth, empathy etc. Case and Dalley's interest here shows the transference and countertransference relationship, as discussed in further detail below.*

Therefore, there are at least two fundamental ways of doing art therapy. Art *as* therapy and art *in* therapy. A different emphasis can be given both to the process of the creation of art, and to psychotherapy. Consequently, some art therapists practise primarily according to the principle that the process itself is the main healing effect, whereas others focus on the therapeutic relationship and the exploration of the meaning of the artwork. The artists among us would certainly emphasise the healing power of the art process 'art as therapy'. The psychologists among us would probably see it as a tool to facilitate communication through unconscious material. Some might even think in a more contemplative or so called 'transpersonal' way about art therapy connecting us to a deeper and meaningful place that reaches beyond us. Most contemporary art therapists, however, believe that both forms belong together; they influence each other in a meaningful way. Depending on the individual clients and their problems, the emphasis can change from one focus to the other. As practitioners, we can harness the legacy of last century's psychotherapy frameworks, contemporary brain science, and innate human drives to communicate inner experience and creativity, to deliver powerful, transformational therapeutic experiences.

Art 'as' therapy: In this case drawing, painting or sculpting are the main focus. The therapist can also ask the client how he or she feels while doing the picture. **This is for me, more about the process and not as much about the content of the picture!**

'Art as therapy' can be understood as the process of drawing and asking about the process; asking how the client felt while drawing. This is a very important part in art therapy; often, an innocent moment can lead to great insights, a shifting of unconscious to conscious through creative expression and its reflection. If a client is struggling with finding words, art as therapy can become the main approach. This is often favoured in work with clients who have intellectual disabilities, who are very young or elderly, or clients with speech impairments. Immature and novel art therapists often find it easier and less overwhelming doing art as therapy for several years before moving into the more clinical realm of art in therapy. Having said that, art as therapy can also be quite complex and challenging, considering the tasks at hand. Choosing the right materials, for example, or the right activity and being faced with a process that is driven by someone who is not well.

Physiologically or medically speaking, we can find several health benefits for our clients through art as therapy, similarly to meditation. Researchers found a rise of alpha wave pattern, typical of restful alertness, a relaxed state of the mind (Bolwerk et al., 2014). Furthermore, serotonin levels also appear to increase, alleviating the feeling of depression (Malchiodi, 2007). Art making also seems to be beneficial in reducing a person's cortisol levels (Kaimal, Ray & Muniz, 2016), a hormone that the body produces as a response to stress. These are only a few of the benefits that have been widely researched, but of course, there are many more.

Art 'in' therapy: The therapist works with the client to explore the content and the deeper meaning of the picture. We do this by asking the client to **describe what he or she sees in the picture**. It's not about what the art therapist sees in the artwork. It's not about the clients' conscious interpretation either. It's about what is actually there, what they have drawn from their unconscious and how that is then interpreted by the client, for what it is, not what they think it is.

During this gradual process the therapist asks the client to describe their picture in detail. The questions help the client to give descriptions about the picture they have drawn. While clients are looking at their picture and relating to what they see, they can find important insights about their lives (Betensky, 2016). Most analysts would see free association as the key to underlying messages. Similarly, art therapists use pictures as the representation of free associations (Rubin, 2016b), to better understand a client's underlying problems. Through the process of describing the different elements of the picture, the client makes free associations between the images on the page and their own unconscious material. A kind of spontaneous connection occurs between the elements of the picture and the client's unconscious mind, where the visual image is interpreted by the unconscious as a sensation, a memory, or any number of things that are relevant to the client, which then becomes conscious. Once it is conscious it might then be possible to be described in words.

I see an important role for the therapist who relates the information back to the client, using the client's words like a mirror, without projecting their own perception. When the client hears their very own words or descriptions of what they have seen in the picture, repeated by the therapist, it becomes objectified for them. They are able to see their inner self, outside of themselves.

In my experience, however, seeing is often not enough, especially if the client isn't able to interpret. Clients look at their own drawing, but they don't always seem to understand how these colours, shapes and lines relate to them. If the art therapist, however, verbalises the picture giving a description back to the client within the context of the clients' life, then clients are able to reach deep insights into what is really happening for themselves, in their own thinking and in their lives. This will be explained in more detail in the following chapters.

This approach is far more complex than art as therapy and requires good listening skills, and a non-judgmental stance. It calls for a solid understanding of psychotherapy and mental health, but also great intuition. We are not following a 'medical' model here. We can remain open to the unexpected and also trust our 'gut feeling'. Since research indicates that there are neural networks in our gut (Siegel, 2017), creating a 'second brain', it can be seen as good clinical practice to follow our 'gut feeling'. Consequently, the therapist needs to be astute to emotional changes as the client describes their image. This is a key to achieving deep insights in therapy in general. When these changes occur in the client it is good practice to ask appropriate questions. For example, "I am noticing that this is upsetting you", or, "What is going on for you right now? What are you thinking, feeling . . .?"

Look for unique words. If a client says ". . . happy" you could ask, "What is happy for you?" Try to avoid the word 'why', as it encompasses too much. All the answers are in the picture as the unconscious always projects into the picture.

Try to connect with the client as well as you can so they can trust you, feel safe and can answer from the unconscious. If you do this well, their suffering will hopefully transform into compassion for others and a deeper wisdom about life.

Art therapy empowers people. It is, to put it simply, ". . . turning shit into gold," or ". . . turning manure into something that keeps growing and becoming stronger and more beautiful than ever predicted". 'Gold' and 'growth' is the aim of art therapy.

In long-term art therapy, you could also attempt to work with transference and countertransference relationships within this approach. However, this requires a lot of skill and training. Prochaska and Norcross (2013) recommend processing the therapeutic relationship, as dependency often develops, only for longer-term therapy. In transference, the client transfers a significant other person in their life, like the mother, onto the therapist and then sees him or her as such. In countertransference, the therapist transfers a significant other onto the client. If this is processed skilfully, the feelings in the therapist can be used as an indicator as to the kind of emotions the client could also bring up in others, rather than the therapists own issues getting in the way (Case & Dalley, 2014). I can see the benefit of this approach, having grown up with a psychoanalyst mother, but I can also see how this might be quite difficult for new therapists with little training and experience. This can be difficult for those who don't know themselves well enough and suddenly end up in the 'mother or father role' or develop strong feelings towards the client and have no idea what to do about it.

Interpreting

Most clients, sadly enough some practitioners as well, believe that therapists working with the unconscious should interpret the client's associations in talking therapy, or the pictures in art therapy. I have come to the belief that art therapy is more effective and it is more respectful if we allow the client to take the lead and to give meaning to what comes up for them. Part of my reasoning for this is that when a client comes in for therapy, they often want to understand themselves better. They want insight into their internal conflict and emotional challenges, even though they might be experiencing external drama; often, the client is a mystery to themselves. As therapists, by assuming that we have all the answers, that we can analyse a client's pictures and formulate a hypothesis that leads to a resolution of the problem quickly, we cut ourselves off from the journey of true knowledge about the client. It is truth that both the clients and the therapists are seeking, and it has to be uncovered, through a process of the clients understanding their unconscious to some extent. After all, they have to get back to life and hopefully use what they have learnt about themselves in therapy to guide them. If we allow our clients to find their own answers during therapy, then we show them that they can trust in their own self-knowledge and insight. We don't support their bike like dad or mum used to do; they ride it themselves after mum and dad have trusted to let go. On a conscious level, a client can be muddled and confused, depressed and angry and unable to resolve any of their problems, but on an unconscious level there is a lot of wisdom in our clients.

To be fair, this approach might not always work, as some clients may want a more directive approach and expect active interpretation and advice. Moreover, some are not in the position to reach down to their 'inner wisdom', as they are deeply troubled, perhaps experiencing a psychotic episode or having suicidal tendencies. Despite these exceptions however, in my experience, most clients are deeply touched when finding their own answers and a permanent transformation or change is more likely to occur when the answer comes from within rather than from somebody else, regardless of how much of an expert the therapist is.

Even early psychoanalysts including Freud used methods that gave the client a way to interpret their own machinations of behaviour, for example free association; how a person responds unconsciously by associating a word to another word or picture (McWilliams, 2011). Salvador Dali, the great surrealist artist, was known to have used Freudian theory to analyse his own paintings and to better understand his own unconscious (Sutton, 2014).

So it's important to remember that we do not interpret – the client does. This can be quite difficult for the trained psychologist whose job it is to hypothesise, argue, couch and suggest solutions. Although it can be tempting to assume that commonalities in each individual's pictures represent mental states or issues, it is important not to generalise or be too directive. Rather than interpreting and leading the way, the well-qualified art therapist facilitates a process in which the client feels empowered and comes up with their own insights. As the art therapist, assume you know nothing; the clients are the experts of their pictures. While a symbol such as wings or flying could be interpreted as a symbol of freedom, for your particular client it could mean losing connection to the ground and feeling deeply troubled. In the same way, many people believe black indicates sadness and depression, but for someone else it might represent a happy connection with artistic parents who always wore black. We don't know! We can only know when it becomes an epiphany for the client; when they have an insight and it all starts to make sense to them. Instead of hypothesising and interpreting, I suggest better listening, being patient and allowing the clients to find their own answers. It is actually quite a relief when you don't need to know everything.

It is very important for the therapist to not use value judgments such as 'beautiful' about a client's picture, which for the client, may be about something troubling and evoke great sadness or anger, even though aesthetically it might look beautiful to you. Judgements from the therapist about a client's artwork can block the investigative process. Keep comments curious and neutral – such as, "This is interesting" or, "It looks like you have worked really hard today". We can share the picture non-verbally, aesthetically and psychologically with our clients by showing that we are attentive with an open heart and keen interest (Case & Dalley, 2014) without having to add our own judgment and interpretation.

After reviewing all these fundamentals, it is about time we do some art therapy!

Literature

Betensky, M. (2016). Art is therapy: Seeing. In Rubin, J.A. (Ed.), *Approaches to art therapy: Theory and technique* (pp. 1–14) (3rd ed.). New York, Oxon: Routledge-Taylor & Francis Group.

Bolwerk, A., Mack-Andrick, J., Lang, F., Dörfler, A., & Maihöfner, Ch. (2014, July). *How art changes your brain: Differential effects of visual art production and cognitive art evaluation on functional brain connectivity.* Retrieved 9 May 2017 from: http://journals.plos.org/plosone/article?id=10.1371/journal.pone.0101035

Carnevale, J.P. (2015). *Counselling gems, thoughts for the practitioner.* New York: Routledge.

Case, C., & Dalley, T. (2014). *The handbook of art therapy* (3rd ed.). London, New York: Routledge-Taylor & Francis Group.

Edwards, D. (2004). *Art therapy.* London: Sage.

Hill, A. (1948). *Art versus illness.* London: Allen & Unwin.

Hofmann, S.G. (2012). *An introduction to modern CBT: Psychological solutions to mental health problems.* West Sussex: Wiley-Blackwell.

Kaimal. G, Ray. K., & Muniz. J. (2016). Reduction of cortisol levels and participants' responses following art making. *Journal of the American Art Therapy Association. 33*(2), 74–80.

Kramer, E. (1971). *Art as therapy with children*. New York: Schocken Books.

McWilliams, N. (2011). *Psychoanalytic diagnosis: Understanding personality structure in the clinical process* (2nd ed.). New York: Guilford Publications.

Malchiodi, C. (2007). *The art therapy sourcebook* (2nd ed.). New York: McGraw-Hill.

Malchiodi, C.A. (2012). Clinical approaches to art therapy. In C.A. Malchiodi (Ed.), *Handbook of art therapy* (pp. 53–140). New York: Guilford Press.

Maslow, A.H. (1968). *Toward a psychology of being* (2nd ed.). Princeton, NJ: Van Nostrand.

Moon, B. (2016). Art therapy: Humanism in action. In Rubin, J.A. (Ed.), *Approaches to art therapy: Theory and technique* (pp. 203–211) (3rd ed.). New York, Oxon: Routledge.

Naumburg, M. (1953). *Psychoneurotic art: Its function in psychotherapy*. New York: Grune and Stratton.

Prochaska, J.O., & Norcross, J.C. (2013). *Systems of psychotherapy: A transtheoretical analysis* (8th ed.). Stamford: Cengage Learning.

Rogers, C.R. (1951). *Client-centered therapy*. London: Constable.

Rubin, J.A. (2016a). Introduction. In Rubin, J.A. (Ed.), *Approaches to art therapy: Theory and technique* (pp. 1–14) (3rd ed.). New York, Oxon: Routledge.

Rubin, J.A. (2016b). Discovery and insight in art therapy. In Rubin, J.A. (Ed.), *Approaches to art therapy: Theory and technique* (pp. 71–86) (3rd ed.). New York, Oxon: Routledge.

Siegel, D.J. (2017). *Mind: A journey to the heart of being human*. New York, London: Norton.

Sutton, A. (2014, October). Art and the unconscious: A semiotic case study of the painting process. Retrieved from: https://lauda.ulapland.fi/bitstream/handle/10024/61720/Sutton_Asta_ActaE_155pdfA.pdf

Swan-Foster (2016). Jungian art therapy. In J.A. Rubin (Ed.), *Approaches to art therapy: Theory and technique* (pp. 167–188) (3rd ed.). New York, Oxon: Routledge.

Tobin, M. (2015, May). A brief history of art therapy: From Freud to Naumburg and Kramer. Retrieved 4 April 2018 from www.researchgate.net/publication/276207648

Trull, T.J., & Prinstein, M.J. (2013). *Clinical psychology* (8th ed.). Belmont: Wadsworth.

Ulman, E., & Dachinger, P. (1975). *Art therapy in theory and practice*. New York: Schocken Books-Chicago.

Waite, M., & Hawker, S. (2009). *Oxford paperback dictionary & thesaurus*. Oxford: Oxford University Press.

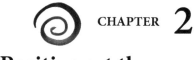

CHAPTER **2**

Positive art therapy

Positive psychology, art therapy and the science of 'happiness' cross paths as they work towards the idea of optimal functioning.

We are living in what is possibly the most informative time in the history of the world, and humans on a large scale can immerse themselves in an enormous amount of information. Technology that can give people immediate results, access to games, recipes, friends, fast communication, entertainment and so much more. And yet this world of play and pleasure, coupled with work commitments and a bucket list of activities, may not be much 'happier' than the world of Socrates (400 BC), one of the first philosophers, who asked the question, 'What is a good life?'

The Pagans used rituals to express their desire for a good harvest. Buddhists practise the principle of 'letting go' in order to achieve inner peace and Christians use prayer. Shamans and healers use chanting as a way of healing the mind and body; all systems of belief for the purpose of making a better life.

As a student of theology, prior to becoming an art therapist and psychologist, I researched many religions that have used different systems to explain how a human being should live, or what a human should think in order to achieve a 'good life'. Although much of this question seems to have an answer in the external, in that human beings can be happy if their comforts and needs are met, a great deal of what makes life worth living is actually dependent upon how we view ourselves and the world. How we feel and what we think.

As psychoanalysts have discovered, thinking is mostly unconscious and the mind, which goes through approximately 60,000 thoughts a day, is likened to a chattering monkey. It never stops thinking. The chatter can fade when the mind is focused on a particular task, or engaged in an entertaining film, but left to its own devices will continue to have a random process of thoughts that seem to come up from nowhere and anywhere. One moment we have a memory brought on by someone wearing perfume, then we remember a fragment of a song, and then the next moment we realise we still haven't finished reading that novel and so on, ad infinitum. All of these thoughts flow like a stream. Whether we are consciously aware of our thoughts or not, they can feel invasive, making us want to immerse ourselves in something to escape our own thinking. If there is nothing to give our attention to, the chatter returns, along with negative thoughts, which can make us feel depressed or anxious. So much for the good life!

When Vincent Van Gogh checked himself into a mental hospital in Saint-Rémy, France, in the late nineteenth century and stayed for one year, he produced more than 100 drawings and around 140 paintings. As is written in his letters to his brother, Theo, Vincent experienced greater life purpose and meaning, and more positive emotions during this period of creativity. Art practice often makes us feel better, even though sometimes it seems to come from suffering. It could well be suggested that Van Gogh's art helped to induce feelings of happiness, a form of 'positive art therapy' that helped him to function.

In the last 70 years psychologists and psychotherapists in general have dramatically increased their knowledge, their understanding and their treatment of psychological disorders. However, by the end of the century, the American psychologist Martin Seligman and Hungarian-American psychologist, Mihaly Csikszentmihalyi (2000) claimed that we knew very little about what makes life worth living. This focus on positive aspects of life started the movement of positive psychology (Gable & Haidt, 2005).

Positive psychology aims to address the imbalance between studies on disorders and studies on what contributes to optimal functioning (Seligman & Csikszentmihalyi, 2000). Advocates of positive psychology recognise, however, that the rest of psychology is not negative, and that distressing, dysfunctional and negative aspects of life can be a reality, and need to be dealt with. The objective is to integrate and complement the existing body of knowledge (Gable & Haidt, 2005). Peterson, Park, and Seligman (2005) claimed that there are several findings that indicate, for example, that strengths of character can buffer against ill health. Although these findings are important, positive health extends beyond the absence of illness (Ryff & Singer, 1998). Therefore, positive psychology attempts to contribute to the existing body of knowledge but with its main focus on optimal functioning, independent of illnesses and disorders. Positive art therapy combines the ideas of positive psychology with the creative process (Wilkinson & Chilton, 2013) and allows for the discovery of strengthening unconscious material.

Inner Resources, our first art therapy intervention in this book, is an exploration of early childhood, adolescence and adulthood to discover what makes us happy in life, and what we might have forgotten that can still make us happy. It is one of the best techniques I have come across and often during the early stages I use it with many of my depressed clients. I have been introduced to this approach by the German art therapists Ludwig Seyfried and Brigitte Held.

Task: early childhood Inner Resources

Time: Allow 1–2 hours for this activity.

Materials to choose from: A4 or A3 paper (printer paper or 'cartridge', which is thicker and heavier paper), colour pencils, oil or soft crayons, water colours or acrylic paint. Also include brushes, cups and a paint mixing board (palette) or empty egg carton.

Spend at least one hour on this task. Try to keep your energy within and try not to talk to anyone during the process. Turn the phone off and other distractions. Put your 'heart and soul' into the picture. Be in the moment and be aware of everything you draw.

Instructions

Draw/paint an experience from your early childhood, when you were three to six years of age. Depict a happy memory, a strong positive experience, when you were in excellent condition, where everything was wonderful, and you felt good and strong. You might have been alone or with others – visualise the environment where you were and bring the experience back into your consciousness. *Note: If you really can't find an experience from your early childhood, you can choose one when you were a bit older, or even a teenager. Don't give up too early. There might be an experience in your early childhood that was absolutely positive.*

Process

When you are drawing or painting your picture, throughout the process, notice your thoughts and feelings. Try to be mindful or 'awareful', i.e. being aware of your current thoughts, feelings and body sensations. Also, try to be spiritually open to your positive experiences throughout the image-making process. Be there, in the moment, as if you are experiencing it in the 'now'. Our unconscious does not understand time well, so things that happened in the past can be as strongly experienced in the present, as if they are happening now. This is often the case for negative experiences like trauma, but generally not understood or recognised for positive experiences. If negative memories come up, try to let them go, visualise them sitting on top of a cloud that passes by, and refocus on your positive experience. This might take several attempts as you work through the process.

Reflections

Reflect on the following by looking closely at your picture and take notes based on the following questions.

What materials have you chosen and how did you feel about the choice? Any hesitation or excitement? Could you start easily, or did you struggle? Did you stay with one material, or did you explore different options? What happened while you were drawing? How was that? Did you experience happiness, bliss or other strong feelings like melancholia or sadness? Did you allow mess to happen, or did you keep it all nice and tidy? At what stage of your drawing did any strong feelings emerge? What were you drawing when you had these feelings? Can you see a connection to your life? What could this possibly mean to you?

At this stage of the process it is just light and playful. Clients often tell me that they enjoyed doing the picture and that's about it. Sometimes, a client might become very teary while drawing a parent, for example, only realising later how much they are missing them.

Look for the positive

Please be aware that it is much easier to remember negative feelings or even look for the negative in the picture, than to experience and see the positive components. In their early childhood picture clients will often see the negative first, e.g. if the father is missing, because he was often away or because the parents were divorced, or he was very aggressive or violent. We tend to be quite focused on the negative. There is an evolutionary reason for this to do with our inbuilt 'flight or fight' response. We are always watching out for danger. The sabre-toothed tiger at the entrance of our cave could have pounced at any time, so we needed this inbuilt response. But watching out for another birthday cake, the day after we have received one, does not have much survival purpose. According to Csikszentimihalyi (2011), our brains are 'hard wired to worry' unless we are focused on other thoughts.

Art in therapy

After we have looked at the process (art as therapy), we can then look at the picture (art in therapy). See Chapter 1 for clarification on the difference between art *as* therapy and art *in* therapy.

Themes and questions

Have a pen and paper handy for notes. Ask the client, or answer for yourself, the following: Tell me about your picture? What is happening? What is the story of your happy experience?

Write down the answers to all the questions above. You could also purchase a journal where you note down your answers and reflections while reading this book. A couple of pieces of paper do the same job, but make sure you keep them together with your drawings and paintings. *Note: You will get a lot more out of the techniques in this book if you always take notes after doing the exercises.*

It's a good feeling . . .

Build sentences related to your picture, starting each sentence with the words, "*It's a good feeling* . . ." Please write them down. Take your time to find meaningful sentences that go beyond, "It's a good feeling to be happy". I often ask my clients, "What is making you happy here?" They might respond, "Being independent . . . doing what I want to do . . . feeling free". "It's a good feeling to be free", might be a more meaningful sentence than just ". . . to be happy", which is less descriptive and less personal. You need to look for relationships like, "it's a good feeling to be close to Mum . . . that she cares . . . that she loves me".

You might have sensed that this technique is similar to how our predecessors, Freud and Jung, worked with free associations. Contrary to common belief, analytic art therapists, psychoanalysts and psychodynamic therapists do not interpret as much as you might think, but facilitate a respectful process where clients find their own answers through free associations and more (McWilliams, 2011; Rubin, 2016). Therefore, when working with clients, please make sure you don't suggest associations, or descriptions, as they are most likely your own projections, which won't help your clients. We are aiming for the deeper experiences and wisdom in our clients. If you understand this now for the first time, you have just made a quantum leap in becoming a good art therapist. It is never about us and how clever we might think we are, but always about our clients and how to assist them in finding their own answers. Therefore, it is sometimes better to know less, and learn to be humble, respectful and deeply appreciative, witnessing what is becoming conscious in someone else.

Senses

Now let's look at some science. Label sensual experiences: taste, sight, smell, touch and sound. Some researchers have found more senses than these five. Interoception, for example, "what we feel from inside our body", mental activities "thoughts, emotions and memories" and "connectedness to others" (Siegel, 2017, p. 229). For this activity however, and for the clients' sake, I suggest we keep it simple.

Look at the picture you have drawn or painted, and think like an empirical scientist. Describe the sensual experience from your picture. Write the main sensual experiences down in great detail, e.g. the ice cream tastes sweet, cold and crunchy. Look for *all* the sensual experiences in your picture and try to find descriptive words for them; make it as detailed as you can. This is not about how you felt in this experience and what it meant to you. It's not about feeling free and appreciating life. We have done this part already. Now, it's about constructing a scientific sensory exploration. I often ask my clients to imagine they are describing the sensation to someone on the phone who has never experienced or seen the sensual experience. If, for example, your friend has never experienced sitting in a tree, how would you describe that experience scientifically? What would the bodily sensations feel like?

Do you have more ideas about your picture? Please add them to your notes.

Delete the descriptions that are just about your feelings or that might have some meaning but aren't sensual. Just highlight the ones that can be described as sensual, e.g. hard and rough to sit on, vanilla sugary sweet, glowing and illuminating everything etc. Delete words like makes me feel free, magical, heartfelt etc.

Link to now

The next step is to do some self-detective work and make the sensual descriptions take effect in the 'now'. What could you do today sensually to give you the same experience? Return to the 'good feelings' from the start of this activity, and from the descriptions you have made, ask yourself which of these sensory experiences can still give you a similar feeling. You will find that some of the sensual experiences from your past are experiences that you still like today. Do you still like playing with dogs, wearing beautiful leather shoes or surrounding yourself with Christmas lights all year round? Why do you like these things? It's more than likely that they remind you unconsciously of your early childhood and the good feelings you have associated to them. *Note: Sometimes my clients, especially those that are depressed, struggle to find links to the present, as they might experience 'everything' negatively. Therefore, I ask them to play being a detective for the next week, try different sensual activities from the list above and see if they can bring back some of those good feelings. Cognitive behaviour therapy works really well here, as we have to plan for some activities that our clients can do and ask them to rate the activities and see how emotional they get. Therefore, we might give them a homework task like the following.*

Homework

In your own time, engage with the sensory experiences you have explored in the 'link to now' section. Each time you engage with this sensual activity, you might experience the happy feelings from the 'It's a good feeling section', even though certain people might no longer be around you or you may have no current affinity with the place or scenario. If this does not happen, keep searching for the elements of the sensory experience, the colours, materials, sounds, tastes, smells, etc. Be a sensory detective and notice the feelings that 'pop up'. You might even feel like rating the different experiences where, '1' is a low emotional response and '10' is high, representing how you felt back in your early childhood and how in the present you can feel when experiencing all those positive emotions.

Therapy

After you have found your personal sensory experience(s) that bring(s) up the old feelings from your early childhood, you are in a great position to make your life more positive and fulfilling. When you are feeling stressed, depressed or just need a break, engage physically (not just mentally) with your sensual activity. Go out into nature, feel the wind in your hair, ride your bicycle or drive your car with an open window, walk on the beach for hours, watch the sun go down with a cup of tea in your hand, etc. The emotional experience of your early childhood, such as feeling loved or free is actually 'anchored' in your senses (e.g. walking on the beach or riding your bicycle). Being anchored is a good metaphor for connecting to something very strong, like the anchor is driven into the ground underneath a boat. By actively pursuing these sensory experiences in the present, you will psychologically re-enact the positive feelings from the past. As we know, the unconscious does not understand time like we know it in our conscious mind, so whatever happened in the past (still in our unconscious), especially strong experiences, can be triggered in the present, (conscious), in this case through sensory experiences.

The link to trauma work

Something very similar happens when we have a traumatic experience. The emotional trauma 'anchors' in the sensory experience of the body. It's as if the body is trying to make sense of the trauma, that this is really happening, and looks for a sensory confirmation. For example, if a person experienced an assault 20 years previously by someone who heavily smelled of garlic, the victim will probably still hate the smell of garlic to this day. Most psychologists are aware of this link, especially when working with patients with post-traumatic stress disorder (PTSD). I have not, however, met any psychologists who knew that something very similar happens with very positive experiences.

The great advantage of art therapy versus the Freudian talking cure is that pictures remain available over time. The significance of the inner story never gets lost, but remains in the picture through different levels of meaning, with some easier to understand and verbalise and others not so (Case & Dalley, 2014). If you choose to have a look at your resource images in a couple of months or years to come, you might even discover something new, surprising and unique to you.

Depressed clients

I use the 'Inner Resources' approach with many of my depressed clients. I have found that they can be so low functioning, that when they come to art therapy I need to 'build them up', before looking at things that might be depressing in their lives.

Most people assume that depressed clients are really sad, but the reality of depression is often quite different. Instead of feeling sad, seriously depressed clients often don't feel anything apart from feeling depressed. They are kind of emotionally frozen, empty, blunt and 'fossilised'. It is a loss of sensual and emotional receptivity and all experiences become narrow, rigid and inhibited (Spreti, 2012). This creates a suffering in the client. When the feeling of sadness returns to these clients, they can cry again. It is actually a sign that they are getting better. They might not experience happiness straight away as they are beginning to feel less depressed, but they might become more open, feel less inhibited, or show signs of inner motivation

I have noticed that depressed clients rarely draw dark depressive pictures, as some people might assume, but contrary to that assumption, they draw fragile, cute little landscapes, with little flowers, or a tiny stream meandering through the landscape. Usually everything is extremely soft, and the textures and colours are very faint and hardly visible. This type of drawing mirrors their experience of not feeling anything, of being 'frozen', or feeling 'dead'. As the art therapy progresses, I have noticed that the textures and colours become stronger, and the colours are more visible and 'make statements'. Overall, the picture gains strength and content, mirroring again the client's personal experiences.

I believe that the job of an art therapist is to give depressed clients some time out, allow them to regress and when they are ready, they can find their way back into the present. Drawing pictures, making sculptures and being creative in any way can help enormously to take the burden off their shoulders and lighten the load they carry around with them. In art therapy, I make sure I keep my timely schedule of activities, so it gives the clients the sense that something is permanent, remembering there is no pressure to participate, only a gentle reminder. In that way, clients can gradually find their way back to work and social activities.

My greatest learning in psychiatry with depressed clients was when I worked with the popular German art therapist Flora von Spreti who advised me not to actively help my clients, but to try to understand my countertransferences (repressed feelings of the therapist aroused by the patient), where I felt I couldn't do anything and was too involved in the suffering of my client. The challenge was understanding my own frustration and even my emerging anger when dealing with depressed clients. She recommended a therapeutic stance of cognitive empathy, where I would not get emotional myself, but remain interested, patient, authentic and show good humour. This has become the baseline of good therapy for me ever since, and the informed reader would have recognised that it is quite similar to the Rogerian client-centred approach.

Early childhood Inner Resources: Emma

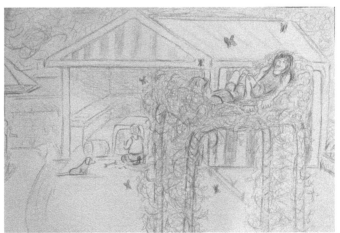

Step 1: Story

Rob: Tell me about your story.

Emma: My art depicts my five-year-old self with my best friend, Adam. Adam and I used to climb the arbour and catch butterflies. Dad was always outside and watching us.

Step 2: It's a good feeling

Rob: Please build a couple of sentences starting with "It is a good feeling . . ."

Emma: It's a good feeling to lie in the lush leaves, to sink into them; it is a good feeling to know Dad is there. It is a good feeling to be with my friend.

Rob: So, it's a good feeling lying in the lush leaves? What is so good about lying in the lush leaves?

Emma: It's a good feeling to be enclosed.

Rob: What is good about being enclosed? What do you feel?

Emma: Hidden, enclosed and **safe**.

Rob: What about your dad? What is the good feeling?

Emma: He makes me feel safe.

Rob: What else makes you feel safe about Dad?

Emma: He is big, strong and always fixes things. He is very **loving**.

Rob: Please use a sentence.

Emma: It is a good feeling to be loved by my dad.

Rob: What are you thinking right now?

Emma: I feel like I am going to cry.

Rob: Is your dad still alive? Do you still have contact with your friend Adam?

Emma: No.

Rob: What did you feel when you recalled this memory?

Emma: I felt safe and loved.

Step 3: The five senses

Rob: What was the strongest sensory experience – lush leaves? What do you still love today?

Emma: Leaves, denseness of the foliage and smell.

Rob: How did it smell?

Emma: Viny; sap coming out.

Rob: Is there something today that brings this back?

Emma: Camping.

Rob: Camping in lush surroundings?

Emma: Yes.

Rob: That's why you like camping; you feel safe, enclosed and loved.

Emma: Very, very spot on!

Rob: Camping is your early childhood Inner Resource. Every time you feel stressed in your relationship, or work, or with your children, etc., go camping; it will make you feel enclosed and safe. You will feel the love of your dad and you will feel you can cope better with what is waiting for you at home or work. Does this make sense?

Emma: Very much. I have actually turned my backyard into a resort. I don't need to go camping. I also go to garage sales every Saturday, and have been going for the past eight years. I buy plants and have created a tropical, camping escape in my backyard.

Rob: Lush surroundings, I love it. I can also see your dad working in the garage in the picture. You have created your early childhood resource in your backyard today.

Emma: When my dad passed away I was depressed – I looked at my paradise but didn't care. Then when I started to feel better, I noted that I went to buy plants and to garage sales, and I knew I was getting better.

Rob: People who are in a bad place, have often lost contact with the things that make them feel good. This is where art therapy can help. When you know what makes you happy through art therapy, you can deliberately do those things in life, and it will take you to a timeless and meaningful place – it is your natural anti-depressant.

Clay work

Another, more tactile, way to engage the feeling of your early childhood Inner Resource is with clay. If you have some spare time, try giving your feelings three-dimensional expression using a mouldable substance such as air-drying clay. This can be art *as* therapy for you.

Further work with Inner Resources

Explore more Inner Resources and beautiful places within yourself in your time-line that can have an enormous outcome in your present life. You might choose to do these activities now or later after reading the entire book.

> Picture 2: Choose a great experience from when you were an adolescent and do the entire process from above using that experience.
>
> Picture 3: Choose a great experience from your time as an adult and repeat the above process using that experience.

An unusual case study with an amazing outcome

A five-year-old boy, Daniel, was referred to me for serious sibling rivalry. He tried to kill his younger brother several times, and had to be supervised non-stop by the time I saw him.

In our first session I assumed that Daniel expected to be reprimanded, as his behaviour seemed quite reticent. I asked him to draw the happiest moment in his life, his 'early childhood experience'. Even though he was still in his early child-hood, having quite a bad time, I felt it was important to find his happiest memory. Daniel drew himself and another larger figure in yellow, lying on a blue watery surface. He described his happy experience as being with Dad, playing in the water and feeling loved. Daniel did not see much of his father, who was often travel-ling on work assignments, and when he was at home, he didn't spend much time with Daniel. As a consequence of being separated from his father, Daniel took to 'naughty' behaviour towards his younger brother.

The following session, I asked Daniel to draw his younger brother, which he did reluctantly. He described his brother in the picture as somebody he 'hated'. I asked him to describe the imagery, for what it looked like, and not what he felt. He said, ". . . it looks like a person lying in the water. The body is yellow, like the sun warming it, the water is cool, like cooling down the body", and then he started crying. I asked him, "What is happening for you now? What is making you upset?" He responded that he did not understand his picture. I prompted him to tell me more about it, and he said he didn't understand why he drew his brother, whom he hates so much, in this way; lying in the sun, in the blue pool, just like he drew himself and his father, last week in art therapy. "Why is this is upsetting you so much?" I enquired. He answered, while sobbing, "My brother looks like me, he is like me, he wants the same things, like me, he wants to be close to Dad". "How does that make you feel about your brother?" I asked, and Daniel said, "He is like me, and I don't want to hurt him anymore".

The following week, his entire family including the father, showed up at our art therapy session. They told me how amazing their week was, because Daniel now showed great interest in playing with his younger brother as he had never done before. When we were alone, I asked Daniel to draw a picture of himself with his brother, and he drew himself on top of an elephant with his brother sitting behind him. I enquired about the picture and he said, "We are on a safari, and there are many dangerous animals around us. Can you see the crocodile at the bottom? The snake in the tree and the tiger, hidden in the bushes?" "Yes", I said and asked him how the two boys in the picture felt. "Great, because I am looking after my younger brother."

This significant transformation really helped Daniel. Fifteen years later, I saw him at a local event, the benefits of living in a small community, and he told me he was studying medicine to become a GP.

Psychologically and spiritually speaking, I see this as a transformation of a victim, who was displacing his aggression towards his younger brother, into a hero who masters his emotions and suffering, and uses his inner strength and power in an integrated way for the purpose to help others.

Working with positive projections

There are many ways of working with positive unconscious content to make it more available to our clients. After exploring our Inner Resources, let's look at a technique that is brief, playful and changes the way we might look at others and ourselves.

Most of us are familiar with psychological projections. These are the negative aspects in ourselves that our conscious mind can't deal with, when we sometimes project onto someone or something else, leaving our conscious mind free of guilt. For example, a woman who gets really angry with her messy neighbour, doesn't realise that she is, in fact, angry with her own physical or emotional mess, or becomes outraged with greedy and egocentric politicians without noticing her own greed and narcissism. Then there is the classic projection where you jealously blame your partner for their flirtatious behaviour when, in fact, you are hiding your own wandering eye. You project an unconscious, undesired emotion from within yourself onto someone else, as if you personally don't possess it.

In positive art therapy, I would like to introduce you to the idea of our inner 'positive projections'. These are not widely recognised or discussed, and I imagine most psychologists are not very familiar with them. The 'Role Models Technique' is a good example for this phenomenon and highly beneficial, as it makes us aware of the positive aspects in ourselves, and that we can consciously generate positive feelings into our daily life.

Task: role models

Time: Allow 1–2 hours for this activity.

Materials: Like above, paper, colour pencils, crayons, paint, etc.

Instructions

Do three separate drawings of three people you admire and look up to (one could be a family member). Draw each person doing the thing you admire about them or what simply impresses you.

Note: This activity can also be done with portraits, but I have found over the years that drawing/seeing the role model doing something, i.e. an activity or work, adds valuable information from the unconscious.

You might be aware of the flaws of your role model as well, especially with ambiguous family members, but try to focus on the positive aspects in this activity. The person you admire can also be a fictional character from a movie, a book, or a person from the past, like one of our great historic figures who made a difference in the world.

Exploration of the role models

Please keep taking notes in your journal.

Who did you choose as your role models? Look at your first picture and describe what you see. How have you represented him/her? What is he or she doing?

Key questions:

- What are the characteristics (qualities you admire) of this role model? Try to find at least three and write them down before you keep reading.
- How do these characteristics relate to **your** life? Are you aware that these are positive projections and that you possess them as well, to a degree? You have projected onto your role model what you already have within you. You might find that some of these characteristics are strongly represented in your life. You might find that you are similar to your role model to some degree.
- Ask yourself which characteristic would you like more of. Which is the most important one for your life right now?

- Once you have chosen it, draw yourself as you imagine you'd be if you had more of that desired characteristic. Your unconscious will facilitate your progress towards this. Please attend to details, so your unconscious can project into different aspects of your image. For example: a client might draw her role model as the selfless Mother Teresa working in Africa, but the actual picture might show her teaching at her (the client's) own school, selflessly. This is how unconscious projections often work, when drawn into images. They show your true potential or the next step you should take, out of your own inner wisdom. Therefore, she does not need to go to Africa to be more selfless, but can achieve that in her own school environment.
- Repeat this process for the other two role models.
- Compare the characteristics and messages revealed in each of the three role model activities and see if you can find any similarities. If messages repeat, it might be a 'key' message for you.

In positive art therapy, we consciously examine the unconscious mind and deliberately look at the way positive experiences and inner strengths are expressed through our imagery. We can mindfully use these insights in our daily life, giving way to the power of a positive happier self.

Literature

Case, C., & Dalley, T. (2014). *The handbook of art therapy* (3rd ed.). London, New York: Routledge, Taylor & Francis Group.

Csikszentimihalyi, M. (2011). *'Flow' – the key to unlocking meaning, creativity, and true happiness.* New York: Harper and Collins.

Gable, S.L., & Haidt, J. (2005). What (and why) is positive psychology? *Review of General Psychology, 9*(2), 103.

McWilliams, N. (2011). *Psychoanalytic diagnosis: Understanding personality structure in the clinical process* (2nd ed.). New York: Guilford Publications.

Peterson, Ch., Park, N., & Seligman, M.E.P. (2005). Assessment of character strengths. In G.P. Koocher, J.C. Norcross, & S.S. Hill III (Eds), *Psychologists' desk reference* (pp. 93–98) (2nd ed.). New York: Oxford University Press.

Rubin, J.A. (2016). Discover and insight in art therapy. In Rubin, J.A. (Ed.), *Approaches to art therapy: Theory and technique* (pp. 1–14) (3rd ed.). New York, Oxon: Routledge.

Ryff, C.D., & Singer, B. (1998). The contours of positive human health. *Psychological Inquiry, 9*(1), 1–28.

Seligman, M.E.P., & and Csikszentmihalyi, M. (2000). Positive psychology: An introduction. *American Psychologist, 55*, 5–14.

Siegel, D.J. (2017). *Mind: A journey to the heart of being human.* New York, London: Norton.

Spreti, v.F. (2012). Art therapy with depressed patients (trans.). In F.v. Spreti, P. Martius, & H. Foerstl (Eds), *Art therapy with psychological disorders* (trans.) (2nd ed.) (pp. 183–193). Munich: Urban & Fischer.

Wilkinson, R.A., & Chilto, G. (2013). Positive art therapy: Linking positive psychology to art therapy theory, practice, and research. *Journal of the American Art Therapy Association, 30*(1), 4–11.

CHAPTER 3

Representational images, projective drawings and the House-Tree-Person (HTP) task

Throughout history, shamans, priests, doctors and healers have all used creative expression to help people. During the development of psychology in the early 1900s, Freud and Breuer developed the 'talking cure' to analyse the unconscious mind.

In the late 1930s, when the psychologist John Buck could not help a nine-year-old girl with just talking therapy, he asked her to do a drawing instead (Buck, 1992). This encouragement finally elicited speech and he realised that drawing can access information that cannot be reached through questioning alone. Around the same time, the exploration of the unconscious through drawing had evolved into art therapy. Buck's finding and further research into the unique power of drawing led to a manual, a tool consisting of a series of tests called projective drawings, through which the client could project his or her unconscious thoughts or feelings onto paper. The therapist could then assess aspects of the client's unconscious mind. This was a pivotal moment in history when psychology befriended art and helped to create art therapy as we know it today.

John Buck's House-Tree-Person theory consists of the drawing of three main objects on three separate pieces of paper, a house, a tree, and a person (Yu et al., 2016). Each symbol is believed to represent different core aspects of the individual in therapy. Buck (1948) believed that the house represents the individual's interpersonal relationships, the tree is a symbol of how resourceful one is in their environment, and the person in the picture signifies the individual's perception of self, how they identify themselves and how they function in their environment.

In different approaches, like the Synthetic House-Tree-Person Method (S-HTP), images are drawn on the same page (Fujii et al, 2016; Kato & Suzuki, 2015). In the Kinetic House-Tree-Person method (K-HTP), a certain action is involved in the drawing. This saved time in therapy and also consolidated the interaction and integration of the three components (Li et al., 2014).

The placement of items in a drawing on a page can unintentionally reveal information about the client that they may not have otherwise revealed in a verbal manner, such as the client's social status (Kim et al., 2008). In further studies, Torem et al. (1990) found a correlation between the number of distinctive marks that were drawn onto the tree and the extent of the individual's physical abuse and trauma. This indicated that, although the tree is an inanimate object, individuals will draw this symbol in a way that suggests they can emotionally identify with it (Torem et al., 1990).

In earlier studies it was shown that a client's use of colour in drawings is able to predict different personality aspects, although it was stated at the time that these theories would be difficult to prove (Marzolf & Kirchner, 1973). In addition, a drawing has the potential to have different meanings as it is dependent on the personal, emotional and mental circumstances of the individual. Factors concerning an individual's nationality and culture, as well as their educational background, can modify the meaning of a symbol (Kim et al., 2008).

While many art therapists and psychologists considered the HTP test as unreliable for revealing or measuring the complexities of the unconscious (Killian, 1984), projective drawings like the House-Tree-Person task can be an excellent therapeutic tool for the assessment and counselling process as shown below. The House-Tree-Person task is still used effectively today, often as a way for the therapist to add to the assessment of the client, allowing the client to talk generally about themselves and make unconscious material conscious.

Your House-Tree-Person task

The aim of this exercise is to demonstrate how to work with figurative drawings including a house, a tree and person, with a client. Eventually, all kinds of representational images, like rose bushes, steep mountains, cats and dogs, etc., can be used. I believe this teaching applies to everything we see in our physical environment, not just a house, a tree or a person, but for simplicity's sake, we focus on those three in this chapter. Try this activity yourself before working with a client.

Visualisation

Find a good spot in a room or outside, sit comfortably and close your eyes; perhaps do some relaxation exercises (e.g. meditate and focus on your breathing). Then visualise a house . . . It can be an old house, or a new house; perhaps a small or large house; it can be very simple or with lots of detail. What is it made of? How many people live in it? Put your house in the environment of your choice: a desert, mountains, the sea, a city or in the country. Next imagine a tree . . . any tree, little or large, with lots of leaves or none. What season is it in? Is it deciduous? Finally, imagine yourself in this picture, not in the house but outside it, so you can be clearly seen. What are you doing in the picture?

The HTP drawing

Duration: 1–2 hours

Draw or paint on a piece of A4 or A3 paper, starting with a house, then a tree and lastly, a person (the whole body), an image of yourself as well as you can, using as many colours as you wish. (If this is a group setting, ask the clients not to talk during the drawing process.) You should spend at least one hour doing this drawing with as much detail as possible. **Our unconscious 'likes' projecting through details that escape our control. Therefore, the more detail, the better.** Try not to draw the house you live in now, or used to live in, or would like to live in. Draw a house that suits you right now, emotionally, so that your emotions can be expressed in the colours, lines and shapes. Do the same for the tree and the person.

*Note: Working with a client, you can introduce this type of activity as early as the first session. It is a great assessment task that adds well to your general assessment, and in my experience, whatever is important for your client will probably come up in the picture. Our unconscious is 'driven' to express what is important, and art is an amazing tool for that. In fact, HTP is an easy way to **quickly** reveal some of your client's deep-seated issues. Even their choice of art materials can tell you something about them! Of course, the client will interpret their own drawing as you note down what they say, as discussed earlier. We will see how this works in detail in the following.*

Questions to ask about the HTP drawing

I would like to focus on this here and in most of my book on art in therapy, as a lot has been written about art as therapy, but very little about art in therapy. This does not mean, however, that the creative process is secondary or less important.

Please answer the following questions and take notes as before:

1   How was the process for you? How did you go doing the picture? Did you become emotional during the making of the picture and what were you drawing at that time? How did you resolve this? Was it easy to finish? How did you feel afterwards? What might the meaning of that be for your life at the moment? Simply speaking, compare your emotions in the process to your life's experiences. For example, the house became too small, I could not get it larger, and I felt trapped. Do you feel trapped at the moment?

2   Let's look at your house in the drawing: Can you describe the house in great detail? Please don't forget to write this down. The key here is to describe what you see and not what you think about it. "It is too small, and I feel trapped" vs "I wanted to make it bigger". Be aware of all the details; what they look like and how they make you feel. What's there? What does the roof look like? How about the windows and the door? What is the connection to the ground like? What's missing? What is emphasised or neglected? Who lives there? Are they happy inside or not? At night, do people visit and how do they feel about your house? How easy is it getting to your house? And so on.

3   Now let's look at the tree in the picture: Look at the tree and ask yourself how it appears? It is (again) about what you have done, what it looks like and not what you have planned to do. Ask yourself and write down: How has it grown and developed over the years? Where did the development start and what

does the bottom of your tree look like? Was it ever damaged? What age is it? What season is it in and how does it make you feel? Does it have leaves and fruits and how many? How does that make you feel? Who waters it? How is it looked after? Does it get enough sunshine? How does it feel in its environment? And so on.

Note: I don't really apply a strategy to my questions, but allow my intuition and especially the responses of the client lead me. If they start getting emotional, I ask more about the part of the drawing that made them emotional. This is often the most important part of the entire process. This process is not about ticking boxes and following a manualised program, but more about listening carefully to your client's verbal accounts and body language. You might have noticed, that I have moved away quite dramatically from Buck's original use of this technique (the House-Tree-Person test) where he tried to assess quantitively and empirically all the aspects from the picture. **I am in a therapeutic relationship here. My assumption is that I don't know anything and what I see matters very little, but I go along with the client's responses. For me, it is not about my own projections or countertransferences, but more about the client's insight. They are the expert.**

4   Now let's look at the person in the picture. Please observe and write down:

How similar is the person to you? What is different and how? How do the clothes and setting express their needs? What about their size and age? What's their favourite thing to do? What's something they do not like? How does the person relate to his or her environment? Is he or she doing anything and what does that look like? What is emphasised or neglected, and how does it feel if that is emphasised or neglected? What does it look like, to you? What else strikes you about the person in the picture? **Please describe the person in detail, taking notes, before you continue reading.**

5   Is there a common theme running through your House-Tree-Person picture for you?
6   If you, as the reader, consulted an art therapist, what would he or she do with this information? First, they might ask you about the process of 'art as therapy' and investigate it, especially if you noticed strong emotional changes while you were creating the picture. Noticing emotional changes in your clients is often the fastest way to reach unconscious material. Second, the art therapist would ask you to describe your 'art in therapy' picture, and write down all the descriptions for further work. What does that further work entail or look like? The art therapist might read the descriptions back to you, of the house, the tree and the person, but relate them to your life. For example, people often describe the house as a place where they feel safe or unsafe and where people live together. Therefore, the art therapist could ask the client about all the descriptions in context with safety and relationships. Have a go, and imagine somebody else reading back all the descriptions to you, and ask yourself how they relate to your life.

Case example: John

House

Rob: By just looking at it, please describe your house, the way you see it in the picture and how it feels to you.

John: It looks simple, small, has a solid and safe roof that keeps out the rain, the elements, and things that could damage it . . . Oh, I have forgotten the door and the windows. I wonder how I can get out and how people can get inside the house in my picture?

Rob: Would you say that at the moment your relationships are simple and few, you have few contacts, but you feel safe and able to keep the people away that might hurt or have hurt you in the past?

Note: I am using the house as a symbol for relationships as supported by previous research and my own experience, but be open for other symbols emerging in your clients. The idea of the house representing relationships is just a working hypothesis, and might not always be the case.

John: How do you know? Yes, I have very few friends at the moment, and I don't even know if I could call them friends, but I feel safe and all the people who used to attack me are no longer in my life.

Rob: I also wonder if you find it hard to understand and get close to others now in your life? (This question is based on the missing door and windows.)

John: That is so true. I have felt like this for many years, and I would like to change it now. Very guarded but not close to anybody.

Rob: How do people get to your house in the picture?

John: It is out in the country, quite isolated, might be hard to find.

Rob: Do you feel that you have isolated yourself and make it hard for people to understand you and get close to you?

John: Yes, I definitely don't make it easy for others to see who I am.

Case example: Steve

Tree

One of my clients was trying to be funny and drew his tree cut down in pieces, on the ground with a chainsaw lying next it.

   Note: In my experience, nothing in an artwork is just funny or an accident or a lack of skill. If this was the case, the client would not mention it. The fact that this client talked about his cut down tree in great detail and became emotional, indicated to me that it meant something.

Rob: Can you please describe your tree in the picture, what it looks like to you with all the things you can see and how that feels to you?

Steve:	Well, I guess, the tree used to be a very strong tree, has a huge base with large roots that I can see going deep into the ground. Then somebody came and chopped it down. (He was laughing while he was saying this.)
Rob:	Would you say that in your development, you feel you have achieved a lot in your life, you have received a lot of support as a child and felt well-grounded in your family of origin? (The roots may represent the family of origin.)
Steve:	Absolutely, how do you know that? I have great parents, and I come from a large family who have been incredibly supportive all my life. Now, my parents have died, and my siblings live in different countries, so I have lost that deep sense of connection to my family of origin.
Rob:	I wonder how the tree felt in your picture when it got chopped down?
Steve:	(Smiling) Well, it probably felt like a big shock to the system, like an assault that must have been terribly painful and led to its death.
Rob:	How does the tree look now?
Steve:	It's dead and nothing is going to grow out of that stump ever again.
Rob:	Do you relate to the experience of being assaulted by somebody, a real shock to your system, a terribly painful experience, and because of that you now feel dead?
Steve:	That is incredible. How do you know all this stuff about me? My partner some weeks ago left me in a rage, I got so mad about it, that I lost the plot at work throwing a printer at a colleague, and got fired as a consequence. Now my ex said that I won't ever see my children again.
Rob:	I got it out of your picture.
Steve:	I only tried to be funny with my picture.
Rob:	What happens in a picture or artwork often happens for a reason.
Steve:	What now?
Rob:	Have you noticed how some trees after a bushfire or after being cut down, change? (This question came purely out of my intuition. I wondered if he could see change being possible after all this.)
Steve:	Yeah, sometimes you can find new growth even though it seems impossible.
Rob:	Can you see that potential for growth in you even though it seems impossible?
Steve:	I like that.

Note: We kept working on the potential of change in the following sessions. I discharged Steve with a new sense of hope after about six months of art therapy, CBT and some other approaches that felt useful.

Case example: Sarah

Person

Rob:	Would you mind trying to describe your person in the picture, not what you were thinking about her while you were drawing, but more what she looks like in the picture now and how that feels to you?
Sarah:	She looks happy.

Rob: How can you see that by looking at the picture?

Sarah: She is smiling, kind of, and she has long hair like me, brown with a pink bow at the front. I can even see the freckles on the nose like I have and my large golden earrings.

Rob: What else do you see?

Sarah: Oh, I ran out of time to draw the arms and legs, because I wanted to spend more time with my house that looks really lost in the big forest.

Rob: How does the person in the picture feel about not having arms and legs?

Sarah: Without legs, she probably can't get anywhere, stuck and lost. Without arms, I imagine, she would have great difficulty in achieving anything in life, can't do a thing, poor thing.

Rob: Do you feel at the moment that you can't get anywhere in your life, you feel a bit stuck and lost and also have great difficulty achieving anything?

Sarah: Wow, I haven't told you much about my life yet, as we have only been discussing the children, but that is so true, what you are saying about me. That is exactly how I feel at the moment. I keep telling everyone that I am OK, but I am definitely not. I do feel lost and don't know what to do with my life.

Note: As you can see from these Q&As, clients often realise what is going on for them when they hear back what they have been saying about their picture and putting it into context with their own life.

Theoretical origins of HTP

The HTP technique is founded primarily on personality theories (think about individual differences and commonalities, e.g. the Freudian psychosexual stages of development). A second framework informing its use is 'projectives' (where inner needs and feelings are unconsciously projected into the images of the house, the tree and the person).

Both personality theories and projectives originate in the psychoanalytic and psychodynamic tradition. It is believed that the house, the tree and the person serve as a canvas for aspects of the inner world and personality strengths and weaknesses. John Buck, the founder of the HTP projective drawing task, says, "You may ask, why a house, a tree and a person, and not something else?" (Buck, 1992). The answer is that these were the most common motifs used by clients when asked to draw spontaneously. Buck also found that, regardless of the ability to verbalise, most clients were willing to draw a house, a tree and a person. Moreover, for most clients, those drawings appeared to stimulate verbalisation more than any other items. This does not mean, however, that we limit the list, as we can work with any representational image in a similar way.

Typical issues and populations

The HTP test is often used to detect and gauge child sexual abuse, self-esteem, social competence and many other personality characteristics. John Buck (1948, 1992) believed that the test (not the counselling approach I have used above) was so declarative that he would take any damage on the tree trunk as an indication of when a person had incurred crisis. There is, however, a big question mark as to how effective it is for assessing those criteria.

For now, we will use this technique as a 'tool' to inform an optimal evidence-based intervention and maximise probability of therapeutic efficacy by revealing some of the psychodynamics of a client's personality. HTP may tell us what kind of personality a person has, which strengths may be harnessed to support the treatment and which weaknesses may hinder progress. In an initial session, it is a gentle way to engage and to begin to discover what is important to that person. Think of it as a platinum frequent flyer card – whisking you both past the airport crowds and queues. Getting past the distracting information that can obscure important factors, especially as rapport is being built between you and the client.

The HTP test is a projective technique that may also introduce the client to their inner needs and foster awareness for them, with the therapist as a witness. It can also be used to quickly reveal what the client is focusing on or worrying about. When used by a clinician, like a psychologist, it could be employed to tap into unconscious levels of personality, raise consciousness and contribute to modification of unhelpful thoughts, feelings and behaviour.

The drawings and paintings are viewed as symbolic communications that enable the client to provide their own feedback by reflecting on their images. The client is encouraged to participate actively in the description and analysis of their images in terms of how these relate to their true personality, issues and goals. The therapist's work is to make sense of the images of the house, the tree and the person, as well as the client's responses. Findings should be viewed as speculations or possibilities rather than confirmed facts and should be confirmed by either the client's descriptions and feedback, other background information or other assessments. Once the unconscious meanings of the pictures is known, the client is encouraged to see their thoughts, feelings and behaviours in a different manner.

Limitations and precautions

Art therapists need to be extremely careful not to project their own expression into a client's drawing, but to facilitate revelation of what the client sees and feels. While projective techniques like the HTP drawing are often thought to evade risks such as dishonest compliance (making things up to please the therapist) and are sometimes deemed more candid than structured inventories, the less structured material produces a huge amount of data that can't be reconciled with conventional standards of validity.

I once had a student in my course who drew a red tiled roof, and I asked her to describe the roof. She said it looked "red, warm and solid". I asked how the people who live in this house might feel if they have a roof like this, that is "warm and solid". She replied that she imagined they were "happy, comfortable and connected". I asked her if she felt happy, or had felt happy in the past, or would like to feel happy, comfortable and connected in the future, in her relationships. (Figurative images can be about the past, present or future. This is different for abstract images, which will be discussed in later chapters.) She said that she was very happy in her life, very comfortable with her family and friends and experienced a deep connection, especially to her new husband.

A week later, one of my new clients drew a red tiled roof that was almost identical to my student, so I was curious to know if she felt in the same way. She described the roof as "burning hot" and "about to explode". I asked her how the people who live in this house might feel if they have a roof like this, "burning hot and about to explode". She said they would feel "trapped, probably would like to escape, but wouldn't know how to, would like to call for help, but nobody is there". I asked her if she has ever ". . . felt like this or still feels like this, trapped, wanting to escape, not knowing how, wanting to call for help, but nobody is there?" I added "Did you ever feel like this?" She burst into tears and told me how she was seriously abused as a child, felt trapped, wanted to escape but couldn't find help. As a result she had lost trust with intimate relationships and backs off or ends relationships whenever it gets too close.

This example shows quite clearly, that whatever we see in clients' pictures means very little until we have heard what they see. Let's look at another client, where we go through the entire House-Tree-Person task.

Case example: Natalie

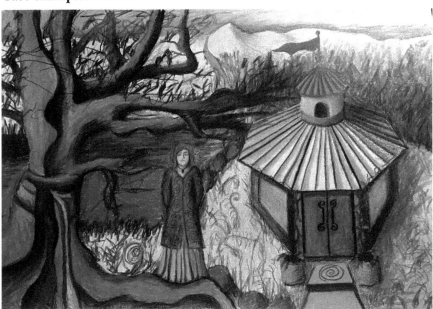

Rob: Would you mind describing your picture in detail?

Note: The following description has been prompted all the way through, but I did not add my questions and enquiries into it, as it would take too long.

Nat: The house is not very big. It looks very small and only a few people would fit inside. It has a hexagonal solid tin roof and on the roof is a circular viewing room where you can see the surroundings with a purple flag on top that looks medieval. It feels protected and safe. The walls of the house have two large windows at the front and this will let in a lot of light. It is a peaceful temple like structure. I am attracted to the door; its colour and shape are very inviting. The house is surrounded by green and is isolated and remote. There are no other houses or people to be seen. I am living there on my own and people visit when invited but it is an effort to get there. The door step is solid and has stepping stones leading up to it and there is a spiral symbol etched into it. The house is made out of wood and tin and is very solid and strong. It is one basic space with no rooms and I imagine minimal furniture. The house is surrounded by greenery and has vines growing up either side of the door. The door handles are an unusual shape, very large and made out or wrought iron. I am happy, peaceful and safe when I am in this house, but I am alone. It is a very quiet place with only the sounds of nature.

Rob: I wonder if you feel that you have only very few close people in your life at the moment? Is protection very important to you, and do you feel safe and peaceful?

Nat: Yes . . .

Rob: Is it possible that people who are close to you are attracted to you and feel invited to get closer? However, you also feel quite isolated at times and alone and if new people want to get close to you, they have to put in quite an effort. Is that right?

Note: These are the only questions that came spontaneously to my mind when I worked with this client. Of course, there are many other questions I could have asked. This is not a manualised treatment program with specific questions, but you are aiming to prompt the client to go deep while trying to understand them.

Nat: Yes, Rob that is correct. I feel close to a few people and don't feel that I need a lot of people in my life to be happy. I need space around me. I feel different and a bit isolated a lot of the time, but have to a certain extent become comfortable with this, as I age. I am in a good place with my life, but it has been hard work, and I believe to a certain extent I will always be working to overcome my issues.

Rob: What about the tree? What comes to mind when you look at your tree in the picture?

Nat: I don't like the tree at all. The tree is large, old, reddish brown in colour and is strangely menacing in appearance. It looks tortured, very hurt, an epitome of pain with lots of shadows. It has struggled to stay alive. The tree has not grown properly, and its roots are partially exposed. Branches have dropped off and are starting to grow again and the leaves on this tree are minimal and struggling to shoot. It is a tree that has leaves all year long, but it appears to be losing its leaves even though the plants around it are green. The tree draws water and nutrients from the river but it's not getting enough sustenance. It gets plenty of sunshine, but still the leaves don't grow. It is ancient and has been struggling to grow for hundreds of years. It is an ugly tree. I can't believe this. I normally love trees. Colourful silk sashes have been wrapped lovingly around the tree to decorate it and make it look less tortured, but they are strangling it. I really don't like it. I would like to chop it down.

Rob: Thinking about your personal development throughout your life, does an epitome of pain come to mind? Feeling tortured and struggling to stay alive? Can you tell me about this? You felt hurt and you could not develop properly and exposed to a degree. Can you tell me about that? You know that you struggled growing up and perhaps still might be, and you feel you don't get enough sustenance to keep you going even though things are much better around you now. Tell me about it. You don't like your past, you feel it's ugly and even though you try to make up for it, you still feel strangled at times by the events of the past. You wish you could just get rid of it, don't you?

Warning: Nat's story is about sexual abuse; feel free to skip the rest of the chapter if you can't stomach it right now. I believe we don't have to stomach everything at any given time.

Nat: Yes I have struggled for most of my life to keep going and have unfortunately attempted suicide numerous times. I have been taking antidepressants, on and off, but not in the last ten years. I hate my past because it is filled with confusion, pain and shame. As a ten-year-old girl I was part of a devoutly Catholic family, and the new parish priest befriended us. From that time on, and for the next seven years, I was sexually abused, almost daily. In the perpetrator's words it was "my fault". I stopped going to church and I would hide from my parents because I felt too ashamed to be in a church. My parents knew that I was troubled by something but didn't know what it was, and I was too afraid to say anything, because I was told by the priest that I would get into serious trouble if anyone found out, and I believed him. I felt dirty and ugly for most of my life even after the abuse stopped. At 17, I became pregnant and the priest forced me to have an abortion. I believed that this was a mortal sin as a Catholic and tried to kill myself. This is when my parents found out. The priest was moved to another parish. It was "hushed up". Nothing was said, it wasn't talked about again, and I continued to live my life of shame. I married at the age of 23, and had two children but by the age of 30, I had a complete breakdown. It took me many years to recover. The priest in question was convicted but let off on a technicality. He was defrocked and died some years ago. I was approached by the

Royal Commission when it started. A lawyer also helped me approach the church directly, and after a lengthy process, I was given a formal apology in writing and compensation. I do feel strangled by the events of the past, and I wish I could just get rid of them. The tree is sick and dying in the picture and maybe this is a good thing if it represents my past, because I will be able to move from it.

Rob: What about the person? What do you see?

Nat: This person is not smiling. She is thinking deeply and trying to detach herself from the tree. She is calm, like a Buddhist, detached. Hands are behind her back and watching, not doing anything. She looks very ceremonious, dressed for a wedding. I am planning to get married later this year. She looks nervous but excited. She looks like she is coming out of the roots of the tree, just hanging on, connected to the horrible tree. She is doing a lot better being calm, not twisted and tortured. She has a nice shape, dressed in my favourite colours, turquoise and purple. I am standing with my hands behind my back looking at the tree and waiting for something to happen. I am looking at the tree, connecting with it, and worrying about it. I have wrapped the tree in colourful silk to make it look better because I really don't like it. It bothers me. I am not smiling because I am trying to decide whether I should chop the tree down or just let it die on its own. I'm worried it will fall on my house. I'm wearing a lapis lazuli pendant around my neck. I wear this often because it is my favourite piece of jewellery. I seem to be standing in the roots of the tree and even though I don't like it I feel some kind of conflicted connection.

Rob: Would you say that you are trying to detach yourself from your past, like a Buddhist, hands behind your back, watching, in a ceremonious dress waiting for your wedding to come, nervous but excited for your life to change? Tell me about it . . . You still worry about what happened to you, and wonder if it will just disappear or if you have to do something actively about it. Make things look better or find a way to get rid of it? It seems you are aware that you are connected to your past and this creates a great conflict for you, is that right?

Nat: At the age of 40, I met a beautiful, intelligent man who understands me and has helped me in my journey to recover. We have been together for 11 years and he has asked me to marry him. This will happen later in the year. I am nervous about it and even though we will marry in the bush and not in a church we will have lots of people at our wedding, and I don't want the feelings of shame to resurface. I worry that I will feel exposed again and am conflicted about being able to have a "normal" happy life in the knowledge that my past is so horrible. However, I feel valued by my fiancé and am hopeful that our ceremony will be special and filled with love. My past does affect my relationships with people, but I will continue to work on myself. I can't change my past, but hopefully I can use it in some way that will be positive. I don't want it to be a destructive influence over my life anymore.

Note: Even though it seems that I am interpreting Nat's drawing for her, I am actually asking questions about what she has told me about her drawing, using her words. She has described herself with "hands behind her back and watching . . . " so I simply ask if she feels as if her hands are behind her back and if she is just watching, i.e. if that is happening currently in her life.

So much time can be wasted in counselling if the client does not really know what is going on for them on a deeper level. The simplicity and the beauty of the HTP technique is that it's a great start to get to know your client, get the conscious expressed, as well as the deep seated unconscious issues into the open, so they can both be addressed in following sessions.

Literature

Buck, J.N. (1948). The HTP technique: A qualitative and quantitative scoring manual. *Journal of Clinical Psychology*, 32, 317–396.

Buck, J.N. (1992). *House-tree-person projective drawing technique (H-T-P): Manual and interpretative guide.* Los Angeles: Western Psychological Services.

Case, C., & Dalley, T. (2014). *The handbook of art therapy* (3rd ed.). London, New York: Routledge, Taylor & Francis Group.

Fujii, C., Okada, A., Akagi, T., Shigeyasu, Y., Shiauchi, A., Hosogi, M., Munemori, E., Ocho, K., & Morishima, T. (2016). Analysis of the synthetic house tree person drawing test for developmental disorder, *Pediatrics International*, 58(1), 8–13.

Kato, D., & Suzuki, M. (2015). Relationships between human figures drawn by Japanese early adolescents: Applying the synthetic house tree person test, *Social Behaviour and Personality: An International Journal*, 45(1), 175.

Killian, G.A. (1984). The house-tree-person technique: Review. In D.J. Keyser, & R.C. Sweetland (Eds), *Test critiques*, (Vol. I, pp. 338–353). Kansas City, MO: Test Corporation of America.

Kim, S., Kang, H., & Kim, K. (2008). Computer determination of placement in a drawing for art therapy assessments. *The Arts in Psychotherapy*, 35(1), 49–59.

Li, C.Y., Chung, L., Hsiung, P.C., Chen, T.J., Liu, S.K., & Pan, A.W. (2014). A psychometric study of the kinetic-house-tree-person scoring system for people with psychiatric disorders in Taiwan. *Hong Kong Journal of Occupational Therapy*, 24, 20–27.

Marzold, S. S., & Kirchner, J. H. (1973). Personality traits and colour choices for house-tree-person drawings. *Journal of Clinical Psychology*, 29, 240–245.

Torem, M. S., Gilbertson, A., & Light, V. (1990). Indications of physical, sexual, and verbal victimisation in projective tree drawings. *Journal of Clinical Psychology*, 900–904.

Yu, Y.Z., Ming, C.Y., Yue, M., Li, J.H., & Ling, L. (2016). House tree person drawing therapy as an intervention for prisoners' prerelease anxiety. *Social Behaviour and Personality*, 44(6), 987–1004.

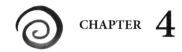

CHAPTER 4

Life Script: Create an alternative script

Sticks and stones may break my bones, but words will never break me.
(**Alexander William Kinglake**)

As we develop through childhood, the words or phrases we hear from our parents, our caregivers and teachers and many others, can affect the way we think consciously and unconsciously. Often, there are statements from those around us, verbalisations that conflict with what we might know to be true from our own experience. People can develop conflicting behaviour, from their own desires, which might be in contradiction with the values they have internalised. So, in fact, words can break us, words and the experience combined, can create intense conflict within.

In the 1950s, Eric Berne, the founder of transactional analysis, researched 'inter' psychic conflicts. These are conflicts between people in their relationships.

This is not to be confused with Freud who was mainly interested in inner conflicts, known as 'intra' psychic conflicts and theorised on three parts of the psyche. According to Freud, the 'id', 'superego' and 'ego' contribute to a person's inner conflict. The 'id' wants immediate satisfaction and is driven by the pleasure principle or child principle: "I want . . . this . . . now". The 'superego' is associated with doing the right thing, evaluating and judging, and has an inner parent voice or societal rules: "No, you can't have this". And the 'ego' or reality principle, seeks a compromise between the 'id' and the 'superego': "You'll just have to wait, be patient or . . .".

Berne proposed that conflicts that clients encountered with others are associated with their 'inner child' (similar to 'id'), their 'inner parent'(similar to 'superego') and their 'inner adult' (similar to 'ego'). Therefore, when we relate to somebody, for example, we might find ourselves talking to them like a 'child', or like a 'parent' or like an 'adult'. They can also choose how they respond to us with their 'inner child', their 'inner parent' or their 'inner adult'.

Messages we receive, especially as children, develop the formation of our 'inner parent'. Our parents might have said things like, "Don't cry, you're a big boy now", or "Act like a girl". The messages we internalise from significant life events can create a life plan, an inner script or Life Script. Men in most societies are often deprived of becoming a nurturing parent or of developing a free and playful 'inner child', so a script may develop for not showing vulnerability or making compromises, which is for 'wusses' under the belief that a man should always be strong, competitive and in control. Thus, the inner conflict is set from a young age.

In my work, combining art therapy with the 'interpsychic conflicts' principle, I tend to use the phrase 'inner wise man' or 'inner wise woman' for the 'inner adult' principle. In the 1950s the 'adult' was considered to be the wise and intelligent man or woman, and because I don't think we have this association any more, I am replacing the term 'inner adult' with 'inner wise man or woman', as the wisdom in us is the key to understanding this principle. One needs considerable wisdom to negotiate the needs of the 'inner child' with the judgmental and authoritarian 'inner parent'.

Example: Imagine, after a very stressful day, asking your partner for a big hug ('inner child') while he is getting ready to watch the AFL Grand Final (annual Australian rules football match) with his friends. He can now respond with his 'inner child' and push you away, saying, "We're watching the game now". Alternatively, he could respond with his 'inner adult' and say, "I have no time for hugs. Please understand that this game is only on once a year". Alternatively, he can respond with his 'inner wise man' and say,

> Darling, I can tell you've had a tough day and need some comfort. As you can see, my friends are all here and the game has already started. Would you mind if I watch the game now? Then after my friends have gone home, I'll spend extra time with you and give you as many hugs as you want. I'll give you undivided attention.

Now, it's up to her to respond to that with her 'inner child', 'inner parent' or 'inner wise woman'.

This process can be used really well in art therapy, where clients come up with different responses and draw them, so the unconscious mind can project how that would look.

Eric Berne explored these interpsychic principles, and discovered that we are strongly influenced in life by 'inner scripts'. A Life Script is a set way of thinking about how we should live our life, often based on decisions made in early childhood, sometimes during adolescence, and even later in life. Often, a rule we give ourselves, or someone gives us after an event or a strong personal experience, can later become our Life Script. For example, your teacher might have said you were no good at maths after you failed to complete a sum, and from then on you might always think you are 'dumb at maths'. The thought is lodged in your mind and will play out in life whenever maths comes up. It's a bit like an inner movie director of whom we are not aware of, sitting in the back of our mind, directing us in regards to what we are thinking, feeling and doing. Our own Life Script is largely unconscious but very influential. It can affect our thinking and behaviour for our whole life unless we can challenge the inner voice of that script, and recognise that it isn't true or doesn't apply any longer.

The psychologist reader might be reminded here of schema therapy by Jeffrey Young. This cognitive approach was especially developed for extremely negative long-term patterns of beliefs and feelings that are a reminder of Life Scripts.

Schemas seem to develop in early childhood and adolescence when someone's needs are not met (Young & Klosko, 1993). When working with Life Scripts in the following, it is useful to ask yourself or your client, what needs were not met and what associated fears are underlying the script or story.

Picture 1: early childhood drawing task

This art therapy technique exploring Life Scripts within art therapy was developed by the German art therapists Ludwig Seyfried and Brigitte Held.

Preparation

You will need A4 (or A3) paper and drawing tools (e.g. coloured pencils, crayons or water colours). Please fold the paper into six segments.

Drawing

- Draw a story with six sequences (can be more, but try it in six). The story is NOT about you, but about someone else. It is a story that you have heard or seen when you were a small child, perhaps four or five years old. This is the earliest story you can remember where something dramatic happened. Ideally something negative or scary that ended well or very badly! It is not something that happened to you personally, it is a story about a character. Perhaps it is a fairy tale, an audio recording, a song, a nursery rhyme, a movie or a good book that was read to you when you were little. The first story that comes to mind and is still very visual is the right one, but please don't choose a 'lame' story where nothing really happens. Our unconscious is created by drama and fear and less by birthday cakes and fairy floss. The Life Script process works with positive stories as well, but is more easily understood through a negative story. As you would need much more experience to work with a positive story, I recommend choosing something more dramatic. If you can't remember anything from a young age, try to recall something from a time when you were a little older. The story needs to have a start, a good story line that develops from picture to picture, and an ending, an outcome.
- It would be helpful for you to have the protagonist, the main leading character of your story, in each of the six pictures, so you don't lose the thread. In this way, we know who the story is about. Please don't draw six different events that are loosely connected to each other, but draw one clear story that develops, for example, "... then Jack got into trouble, because the Giant saw him and started to chase him, but in the end he got away by ... " The story line should be clear, and all the events connected to and leading into each other; it should be sequential.
- Now clear your thoughts and choose one story from early childhood that comes spontaneously to mind – the earliest story that you can remember that was told to you, i.e. a fairy tale or a story from a children's book.
- Take about an hour or two (approximately 10–20 minutes for each picture).

Exploring the drawings

There are three parts that you are required to answer in writing (journal) as in previous exercises: Themes, rules and outcomes. For each part, there are suggested questions and prompts. To explore your Life Script by yourself is an extreme challenge, probably the biggest in this book, but I have supplied enough prompts that should assist you to manage.

The challenge is to bypass your defence mechanisms. I am aware that that is not an easy task to expect from readers when doing this by themselves. If you struggle or don't like the outcome, just skip the task, or ask a friend to read the questions back to you and to assist, or even better an art therapist, psychologist or trained counsellor.

Note: At all times, if you are not well and can't recover yourself, seek help. To register in Germany as an art therapist, we are required to have 100 hours of art therapy. Even if you feel you don't need therapy it is always an advantage to know one's own mind and emotions. It can be a great asset to have experienced the process of psychotherapy before working with your clients.

Themes and questions

Let's start. Take notes now. What is the story about? Tell me about it, picture by picture. What is happening in each of the six pictures? Keep it brief at this stage.

Rules

'You should . . . '

What rules in your story are implied? Please look at each picture, starting with picture one and start with the words "You should . . .", and complete the sentence, addressing it to the protagonist in your story. What do you think he or she should do when you look at picture one? Write it down. What would your recommendations for him or her be if you were to know what is going to happen next? How could he or she prevent something bad from happening? What fear is underlying and what needs are not met? What do you think he or she should do about it? Now ask the same question for each of the following pictures until you get to the outcome of the story. Normally, the outcome does not involve a 'should' message, but rather shows what outcome your protagonist received because of the way he or she was behaving. Most of the time, the last picture or the last two or three pictures is the outcome.

Let's find some further 'shoulds' before we go to the outcome. What does the story teach us? Therefore, "you always should . . ." Is there a moral to the story? Another 'should' that comes to mind? What rule is behind that? Another 'should'?

Outcomes

Now, I would like you to look at the outcome of the story for the protagonist. Normally, the last couple of pictures. What is the outcome of the story? How bad or good is it for the protagonist? I would like you to put it into one, two or three sentences. In noticing these outcomes, try to be childlike and simple. Avoid jargon and diplomatic adult thinking. You are encouraged to be judgmental and to speak from the heart. Also, allow strong emotions to emerge as you describe a time when the world was more black and white, like in a fairy tale. For example, "The outcome is that she finally found real love; a friend for life and lived happily ever after". Or it might be, "He lost his job. Everything he wanted was destroyed and he died a terrible and lonely death". A more distanced way of putting this would be, "She found a life partner and things were turning out okay". Or "He got into financial difficulties, had to deal with some shortcomings and, yes, he died as well". This is what I don't want from my clients Can you see the difference? Turn into a judgmental little child while you are writing your outcomes.

I encourage you not to continue reading further unless you have done all of the above, including the pictures, and answering all the questions in writing.

Your Life Script

This technique is brilliant, because clients are less defensive as they normally don't expect the content of the story to be about them – in fact, they are told that the story is not to be about them. As a result, their defence mechanisms are very low, and they can openly give rules to their protagonist, without realising that those same rules are the ones given to them.

Task: Bring the last two sections together in one sentence in writing, so they make sense. There are two approaches to this depending on whether the outcomes are negative or positive:

- If outcomes supplied by you or the client/are '**negative**' or involve a bad or adverse impact, you can use the following template: *'You should always . . . . (include here all the rules that you have collected above) . . . **otherwise** you . . . (now enter here the outcome of the story as above) . . . '*
- If outcomes supplied by you or the client are '**positive**' or involve good or valued impacts, you can use the following template: *'You should always . . . . (include here all the rules that you have collected above) . . . **only then** you will be . . . . (now enter here the outcome of the story as above) . . . '*

When you have written down the whole Life Script as indicated above, I would like you to read it a couple of times to yourself and see if it 'rings a bell' for you, and if those messages and rules sound familiar to you, in your life so far, or at least for a big part of your life. You might find that some messages and rules are stronger for you than others. Most of my clients follow their Life Script religiously and have a very strong belief that it is good for them to follow those rules.

Sometimes, my more mature students find that their Life Script sentence does not relate to their life any longer, and realise it had a strong influence on them when they were young. For example, ". . . after I have had a breast cancer scare" or ". . . after I got divorced, I somehow stopped following those rules and went the opposite way". It appears to me that when we mature in life, we naturally move away from our Life Script as we are becoming wiser. We also let go of expectations from others and start to follow more of our own heart's desire.

With clients I have not made this observation. I imagine this is related to the fact that they are in great distress, therefore they appear to regress and hang onto old patterns of behaviour and messages that served them well before.

Reversing the Life Script

As it might have become clear, the Life Script created in childhood can be so negative that it has adverse effects on your behaviour later in life. A message may have been given to you when you were very young to keep you safe and healthy, but your early life developed in a complex way that highlighted this message and its demands on you, so you have taken this message to an extreme. Life circumstances have shown you that if you don't totally follow that script, something terrible is going to happen, (negative outcome) or, only if you follow the script religiously, you will end up with your fairy tale happy ending (positive outcome). On a scale from 1–10, you are probably near a 10 following those rules.

I would like to apply the Jungian principle here to the Life Script discussion and propose to reverse it for you by creating an alternative Life Script. You will find this a very helpful format, which you can then use on your own clients. For me, one of C.G. Jung's greatest contributions to analytical psychology was that he saw the world in balance or out of balance, where clients hang on to extreme positions, such as being extremely extrovert or introvert, emotional or rational or animus or anima driven. The skilful therapist now tries to assist the client to move from one extreme position to the opposite position, like a pendulum swinging from one side to the other. The goal, of course, is to achieve a middle position, the number 5 on the scale from 1–10. By the way, the Greek philosopher Aristotle also recommended taking the middle path in life and Confucius also believed that only the middle leads to harmony.

Achieving balance and finding your middle path, can be achieved by reversing the Life Script, and by exploring the opposite of your rules. If your rule was "You should always be safe", then the opposite would be, "Go and get killed". Sounds ridiculous, doesn't it? When we talk about the opposite here, in a Jungian way, we don't literally mean the opposite, but we are looking for a healthier alternative that is on the other side of the scale. Therefore, if your inner message is, "You should always be safe" (number 10 on the scale), the healthy alternative on the other side of the scale, the number 1, might be, "You should take risks".

I have often had students who comment on this and say, "But Rob, isn't it dangerous if 'Mary' is taking risks now? She could get hurt". My response to this is, that most people would probably get hurt when they start taking too many risks, but not Mary, who is a 10 on the scale of being safe. It has become her nature to be safe. Therefore, my underlying goal as an art therapist is not for Mary to really become a 1 on the scale, but to find balance between the extremes. Why am I not asking the client to find a balanced position between being safe and taking a risk and why put them under so much pressure? It is actually quite scary going the opposite way!

Do you know the answer?

The answer is quite simple, and also extremely insightful. If we challenge our clients with a balanced position, like a 5 on the scale, they often won't work hard enough to change their script and end up as a 7 or 8. Whereas, if I ask the client to try as hard as they can to become a 1 in the next couple of weeks, they hopefully move towards the 5, the balanced position, the middle that leads to harmony.

Task: I would like you to go back to all your rules and try to work out the healthy opposite of your rules and the inner messages. However, don't reverse the outcome. You can have a look at the examples below to assist you in your search, but try to find your own version that is unique to you. Some of these scripts might look very similar, but they feel very different for each person.

Case example, Life Script: Jessica

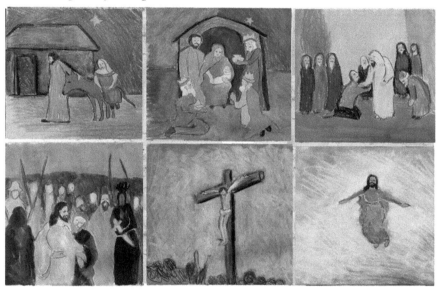

Jessica's story

Jessica is a registered nurse.

Her story is about Jesus's birth, betrayal, death and resurrection. She found strong messages for pictures 3, 4 and 6.

Rules: 'You should'

3rd picture: Jesus is a grown man and is healing the sick – "You should always help and heal others".

4th picture: Jesus is betrayed by Judas and has to run to safety, the tomb – "You should always question others, mistrust them and keep people at a distance", and "You should run away if you don't feel safe, hide and look for safety".

Outcomes: 'Only then'

6th picture: Jesus is resurrected, his body goes up to heaven – 'Only then will you be enlightened, will live forever, be overjoyed, and find meaning in your life".

Jessica's Life Script

You should always help and heal others. You should always question others, mistrust them and keep people at a distance. You should run away if you don't feel safe, hide and look for safety, only then will you be enlightened, live forever, be overjoyed, and find meaning in your life.

Alternative Life Script

I should let others help and heal me and look after myself first. I should trust others and let them close. I should stay and take risks. Only then will I be enlightened, I will live forever, be overjoyed, and find meaning in life.

Note: We keep the same ending of the Life Script and the outcome does not get changed!

Jessica said that she is the type of person who always needs to help, even if people don't want her help. She also told me that she is an expert in running away and doesn't trust anyone. Even though she is in a good relationship now, she does not trust it and feels like running away and ending it. The alternative Life Script makes total sense to her, and it is a relief to Jessica that she can go the opposite way.

Please notice how the second part of the Life Script, the outcome, stayed the same in the Alternative Life Script. This means that the first part of the Life Script was actually a lie and that we only get the good outcome or avoid the bad outcome when we actually do the opposite of what we believe we should be doing. Isn't the work with the unconscious irrational and extraordinary?

Case examples, Life Scripts: Mia, Sarah, Rebecca and John

Note: Pictures have not been added to the stories of the following Life Script examples, but the examples describe how Life Scripts can be reversed into a healthy opposite.

Mia's Life Script

You should always do the right thing, play it safe and seek advice from others at all times, only then will you find resolution, get peace of mind for the rest of your life.

Mia's Alternative Life Script

You should do what you like to do, do unusual things and take risks, and, most of all, follow your heart and inner instinct. Only then, will you find resolution, get peace of mind for the rest of your life.

Sarah's Life Script

You should always push yourself very hard in life, keep going, cope with everything and provide for your family at all times and set things up for their future, only then will you make it to your goal, be cared for by your loved ones and can let go.

Sarah's Alternative Life Script

You should take time out, relax and rest, take time out and take yourself away. You should always allow your family to be independent. You should always trust that the right things will come to you and your loved ones and live fully in the present. Only then will you make it to your goal, be cared for by your loved ones and can let go.

Rebecca's Life Script

You should always keep trying and persevere in life even though you are facing insurmountable difficulties, you should always think about your goal and push through difficulties for a higher purpose and always use your intelligence to achieve those goals, only then you will fall in love, live happily ever after and everything will be well and good.

Rebecca's Alternative Life Script

You should always be flexible and let go of things, be accepting of everything that comes along in a loving way. You should rest as much as you can and enjoy the here and now full heartedly. Only then will you fall in love, live happily ever after and everything will be well and good.

John's Life Script

You should always be careful whom you trust; be especially careful with strangers you don't know. Always be extremely careful being on your own and watch out for danger at all times, otherwise, you will regret it, you will grow old without experiencing your life, without any love, you will get seriously hurt and die a tragic and lonely death.

John's Alternative Life Script

You should always be spontaneous, open to new people in your life, be vulnerable, trust them and allow them to get emotionally close to you. Enjoy being on your own in the moment and do that as much as you can, otherwise, you will regret it, you will grow old without experiencing your life, without any love, you will get seriously hurt and die a tragic and lonely death.

Feedback from clients

After writing the alternative Life Script, I often ask my clients which one looks and feels better and reveals deeper truth for them. They are still drawn to the old version and fearful of the alternative script, but nearly always, they say the second one is the right one for them. This is sometimes hard to explain rationally, but emotionally and experientially it makes absolute sense.

Anxious clients

I have used this approach many times with anxious clients, and I believe it might be extremely beneficial for clients diagnosed with obsessive compulsive disorder (OCD) or clients with similar symptoms.

If we go back all the way to Bowlby's research about attachment disorders, the German art therapist Flora von Spreti (Spreti et al., 2012) indicated that anxiety often has, in its core, a threatened relationship issue. With a lot of adult clients activating situations for anxiety disorders, there are often stress responses about real or perceived separations. Clients with anxiety disorders often depend on others to create security and comfort for them. Sometimes they choose a representational object from home like a comfort blanket or in art therapy a soothing picture that has the same function.

In art therapy, clients can create those objects and manipulate them, work with their need for safety, comfort, and experiment with how much closeness and autonomy they really want and need (Spreti et al. 2012). A topic in art therapy is to address fears and anxieties, so that unconscious resources can be projected and activated, and anxieties producing themes can be understood and finally integrated. Art therapy with those clients is also relationship work in a Rogerian manner (see client-centred therapy).

Surprisingly, the images of anxious clients are not always dark and sinister. Initially, I have noticed, they draw quite beautiful pictures of heavenly environments where everything is fine and wonderful. Sunrise or sunset themes are very popular, opposing their anxiety-provoking situations. As they feel more comfortable in art therapy, the content of the image might change into darker topics, sometimes a dark vortex, a black hole or spiral that is 'trying to suck them in'. Clients and artists often can't find words for their very real experience of deep 'angst'. These kinds of pictures, produced from deep or dark emotions, need attention and involvement, where the facilitator firstly allows pictures like this to happen, but at the same time also helps the client create places of safety. For example, we can propose to create a place that opposes the black hole, or we can ask the client to work with the spiral but bring colour into it (Spreti et al., 2012). In this way we allow integration, and also help the client with their fears of the future, which overwhelms them in the present. Consequently, the main topic for working with anxious clients is to stabilise them, gradually exposing them to their fears while assisting them to feel safe about what is 'scary' and 'unbearable' in their lives.

I normally use the Life Script work with clients who have a very strong 'black and white' thinking and feeling pattern, i.e. only if I clean my hands thoroughly, will I stay alive, or if I don't listen or follow other people's advice, will I die a terrible death, or end up lonely and forgotten. I have found this kind of thinking occurs frequently with clients who have obsessive compulsive disorders (OCD), but also in others with similar mindsets and strong anxieties.

After doing Life Script work with a client, I often received feedback that it was very challenging at the start, but as the client went with the alternative Life Script, it started to free them up. It was often expressed as "... this huge burden was lifted from my shoulders". Interestingly, well-meaning partners of clients often reported that they knew all along that the alternative Life Script was the way to go but, their partner, "... didn't listen to me". Clients, I guess like most of us, find it really hard to take advice from their partners, but are more likely to allow themselves to change in therapy.

Further elaborations for the work with clients

It is the client's story

- Go with the client – don't bring your own prejudices and expectations into it. Allow the client to explore the picture – you will not necessarily understand what the client has drawn or is trying to illustrate.
- It doesn't matter if they get the story wrong, or change the ending of a widely known story. It is what they say that counts, e.g. ending *The Little Red Riding Hood* story with the wolf eating the girl. It is the client's story. The way they have internalised it gives meaning to them. It is not about right or wrong.

Probe until you hit the emotion

- Keep questioning until you get a sense of emotion or pick up that the person resonates with that answer – a gut or intuitive response that you have might engage the emotions and disengage the conscious control.

Note taking

- Make sure you keep an accurate record of the exact words that the client uses. You might need to interrupt the client in order to catch up so that you can get the exact words, but try not to interrupt the flow if possible. Free association needs to be free and uncensored.

Basic premise

- The Life Script is always negative in a way. Holding fast to Life Scripts always has a negative influence on your life – you expend energy maintaining your Life Script.
- This even applies to positive Life Scripts that only have positive messages. I frequently wondered what to do here, but the moment I encouraged the client to look for the healthy alternative, it often started to make sense.
- The Life Script limits our choices and freedom to choose in our present circumstances, not past conditioning. Basically, it is too extreme.

- You take on board messages when you are very young – at first, they may be helpful and beneficial to protect you from danger. Now in the present, you act on past instructions and restrictions. The Life Script becomes a domineering influence on your life. It is your programme that you follow without conscious awareness. To some degree this is OK, as it will keep you functioning and protected.
- However, for some clients they overdo fulfilling the programme. They do not have valid present choices. They are so afraid of what they believe will happen that they are not free to make alternative choices. The choices are reduced by fear.
- To have a wide range of genuine choices, you must have freedom to make 'wise' choices – not ones made by an inner 'child' and inner 'parent'.

Role of the therapist

- As a therapist you **do** have control over how deep to go with your client. You have to take it slowly and see how much the client wants to investigate and reveal.
- Look for body signals. If the words trigger a body response (e.g. tears, catches in voice, shift of posture) **explore what is happening for your client right now** and don't move on in your agenda. This is the best time to make the unconscious conscious for your client. If you miss this moment by being too focused on your own stuff, you might miss the most critical point of this session with your client.

Further Life Scripts

You can do these tasks now or after finishing the book, come back to them.

Picture 2: Adolescence

Preparation

You will need A4 (or A3) paper and drawing tools.
Fold the paper into six segments.

Drawing task

- If you are interested in going further with this activity and have some spare time, you can draw another story with six sequences. Now we are looking at your adolescent Life Script after we have done your early childhood one. This story should once again NOT be about you. It is to be a negative or scary story you remember from your adolescence (approximately 13 to 20 years of age) with a good or bad outcome; a story that influenced you or was important to you in some way; a story that had a huge impact on you; a story that you can remember easily and you know how it started and how it finished. It can be a book, a movie, a play, etc.

- Take about an hour or approximately ten minutes for each picture. You can take longer if you wish, as you do this at home.

Picture 3: Adult

Preparation and drawing task as above if you have lots of spare time, but choose a story this time from your adulthood, from the age of 21 until today.

Exploring the drawings

Explore both **Picture 2** and **Picture 3** as you did for **Picture 1**.

The final overall Life Script

- Look at your picture stories, find common themes and name them. Are there the same or similar messages and rules? What are these? Please write them down.
- Look for common words or synonyms – include them.

If you find that some words come up in two or three Life Scripts, that seem to have a very important representation in your life, then they are probably influencing you in a negative way. It is useful to look for similarities in your client's pictures over time and explore the pattern of behaviour (Betensky, 2016). If the same script sentence comes up two or even three times, there appears to be a greater strength of that message. Remember, Life Scripts are not good for you, especially if the message is repeated over and over again. Therefore, doing the opposite of those rules is going to be even more important for you.

Literature

Betensky, M. (2016). Art is therapy: Seeing. In Rubin, J.A. (Ed.), *Approaches to art therapy: Theory and technique* (3 ed., pp. 1–14). New York and Oxon: Routledge-Taylor & Francis Group.

Spreti, F.v., Martius, P., & Foerstl (2012). *Art therapy with psychological disorders* (trans.) (2nd ed.). Munich: Elsevier/Urban & Fischer.

Young, J.E., & Klosko, J.S. (1993). *Reinventing your life*. New York: Dutton.

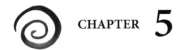

CHAPTER 5

Goals: Overcome obstacles

Our understanding of achieving a goal is usually connected to a practical accomplishment. Most of us are driven to achieve in some way or another, unless we have very little motivation. But even then, we quietly dream of what we want, or who we want to be, where we want to go on our next holiday, or when can we find the time to pursue the goals we truly want. Having desires is not the same thing as setting well planned goals. Sometimes we can end up with an endless list of goals that we can't fulfil, leaving us confused and directionless. Or we can't achieve our goals if they are too far-reaching or completely unrealistic, so then it's back to the drawing board. Most people struggle with goals at some point in their lives, and as our life changes over time, and we change, this in turn affects our goals. There is often a need to set new directions, and look at what our heartfelt goals might be. It's important to spend some time looking at how to achieve them, as well as the obstacles that might be in the way.

A spiritual or holistic goal that involves different aspects of our true needs, is more than just a visible outcome. It can be more authentic in its pursuit than just ticking a 'to do' list. For example, making peace with a neighbour, or even making a new decision to be a more caring person is a spiritual and holistic goal. A change of direction to create more peace in your life, or checking in as to whether the direction you've taken is actually right for you, are also goals. It is not merely about measuring and accountability. It's also important to find out if we truly do desire those far reaching goals, after all, there could be a reason as to why they seem important to us, but we somehow never manage to work towards them. Perhaps there is a goal that is within us, that is far more beneficial to our life and development, which we still need to discover.

If you see a psychologist or a life coach about a goal you have, they might use the S.M.A.R.T. goal-setting strategy, which was originally developed for managers. It is a process that, after brainstorming and identifying your goals, you then decide on a specific goal. The counsellor might assist you in clarifying the goal and check if it is 'S' (specific), 'M' (measurable), 'A' (achievable), 'R' (realistic) and 'T' (timely or track-able). This approach has a very strong cognitive behavioural focus. In art therapy however, we work quite differently. We focus mainly on inner goals and what comes out of the unconscious. When we have uncovered those, however, cognitive behaviour therapy (CBT) might be a good strategy to use afterwards, including S.M.A.R.T., to consolidate the new insights. This is how I mainly use CBT as an art therapist.

Goals

This art therapy process looks at achieving one's goals through integrating what we unconsciously know about our true heart's desire. Our conscious mind will often desire something that deep inside us we don't believe we can achieve because too many obstacles are in the way. The following 'Goals' technique will take us beyond words and return to words, where our unconscious mind will indicate, through our imagery, how to overcome obstacles and truly achieve these heart felt goals.

Goals: drawing task

*The task is to draw three pictures (**figurative and not abstract**).*

1   **Draw a short-term goal that you have at the moment** – something you want to achieve in the next couple of months; perhaps the next step in your life. Draw yourself clearly achieving that goal.

- **Focus on one goal only in your drawing**. If you can't choose between two or three goals, draw more pictures, but please don't put them all in one picture, as you would lose unconscious detail for each of the goals if you pack them all in one picture. 'Art in therapy' needs detail in the images, so you don't run out of unconscious information too quickly. This is like a client in psychoanalysis who is only freely associating for ten seconds versus ten minutes.

- Draw a goal or plan that you would like to become a reality – a dream; a wish you'd like to fulfil; a decision you would like to make. It may be related to your alternative or new Life Script from one of the previous chapters, regarding relationships or your work. What are your priorities? What is really important in your life at the moment? What can you achieve in three months' time that is important to you?

- When drawing, make sure to work **mindfully**, not in a careless or an emotionally detached way. It's about putting your heart into it as well, taking time, and putting as many details in the picture as you can, i.e. drawing yourself with everything else around, including what you are doing and the details of the setting, like the background, the colour of your clothing and more.

- Try **NOT to use symbols or words** i.e. drawing 'love' by using the shape of a heart or writing the word 'love'. This will limit what can be explored out of your unconscious. The symbol and the word are mostly conscious representations, and what we are trying to find here is unconscious projections. There is a role for symbolic representations and words in art therapy, but not here. Far more information is gained when you express love in other ways, i.e. holding hands, sitting together, body position, giving flowers or chocolates or a good book to your loved one, for example.

2   **Middle-term goal picture** – something you want to achieve in two to five years' time. Please draw this on a separate piece of paper.

3   **Long-term goal picture** – something you want to achieve in the next 10 to 20 years. If you are very young, you can choose even 30 or 40 years ahead, the time when you'll retire or reduce your paid work load. Please draw this following the same process as for the previous goals.

Working with the pictures

Please take notes as before to get more out of this exercise.

Themes and description

- In one or two sentences, what is your short-term goal? Please write it down.
- Describe the themes, topics and ideas expressed in the picture.

Note: We'll return to your picture after a relevant case study that will set the scene for what is to come.

Case example

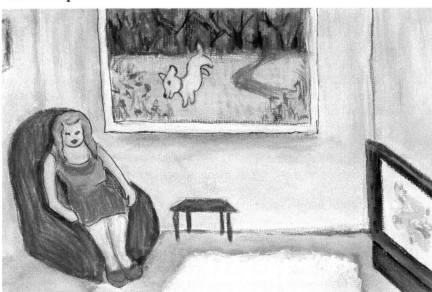

Jennifer's goal

I had a client a couple of years ago who was diagnosed with severe depression and after six months of art therapy she came out of her depression. In our last session, when I planned to discharge her, she asked me if I could do one more thing for her – if I could help her lose weight, as this often contributed to her depressive episodes in the past. She was very overweight. I informed her that as a psychologist I could use the S.M.A.R.T. approach with her (see the beginning of this chapter), involving brainstorming and working on a concrete plan, perhaps with the support of a dietician. The plan could possibly include a change of diet, set meals, regular exercise and going to the gym three times a week. I knew she had a gym membership, even though she 'hated' going there.

Alternatively, as an art therapist I could work with her unconscious and find out what was really holding her back from losing weight and how she could overcome this obstacle. I discussed the goal activity that I have done with some of my clients in the past. She was very interested, since she had consulted many dieticians, tried many diets and had been a member of a gym for years without any success. So, she chose art therapy to lose weight. I informed her that art therapy is not a magic wand, but there might be a good chance she could work out what was holding her back, and how to overcome it. She agreed to 'give it a go', so I asked her to draw a goal picture for the following week, showing how she would look in a year or two, having lost significant weight and doing whatever she believed would help her lose weight. This was not a short-term goal, but more a middle-term goal (see below).

She returned the following week with her picture and showed it proudly to me. It showed her sitting in an armchair in the left-hand side of the picture and on the right-hand side was a TV playing. In the middle of the picture there was a large window that showed the garden outside. There was a path in the garden leading into a forest and a little dog outside that was jumping up and down in front of the window. When I asked Jennifer to show me how she was losing weight in the picture, she told me that she was jogging three times a week along the path that led into the forest and to the gym nearby where she would do more exercise.

Evidence

Questions to ask: What is actually in the picture? What can you see? Are you actually achieving your short-term goal in the picture? In the picture, are you actually doing what helped you to achieve that goal? Can you find evidence that supports that in the picture?

This part is often quite revealing and surprising. I have adopted this idea of looking for evidence from cognitive therapy, and I have found that many of my clients tend to see themselves achieving their goals through their inner eye but, in fact, in the picture they are not! For example, a client once said that the goal in her picture was to have found the love of her life, to have somebody close to her, but in the picture, she was actually gardening alone and there was no indication of a partner. When I asked her where her partner was, she said, "he is on the top of the page, at the road intersection waiting for the bus to go to work". Then I asked her what evidence there was that this was actually her partner and not just anybody waiting for a bus. At this moment, she realised that there was no evidence and that she actually struggled with letting anybody get close to her. This dialogue shows that we often have quite clear ideas about what we want to achieve, and sometimes even very strongly believe in achieving our goals, but our unconscious knows us better, and projects into the artwork what is more likely to happen.

Back to case example: Jennifer's goal

If we look at the previous case of Jennifer and read the last part, you might have noticed that, although Jennifer said she was jogging in the forest to lose weight, she was actually sitting in the armchair watching TV, in her picture. In my experience, this is quite common. The client thinks she is doing what she is supposed to do, not noticing that in the picture her unconscious shows a different scenario. It is called the unconscious mind for a reason, and the significant thing about art therapy is that the client and therapist can actually 'see it', when the evidence becomes clear. This process is very different to normal counselling and the so-called 'talking cure'. It means the art therapist can check in with the client about the discrepancy in the picture, and in Jennifer's case, I could enquire if she was really running in the picture or not. Jennifer said she was. However, she still couldn't see that she wasn't. So, I continued questioning her. I asked her if she could show me where she was running in the picture, because I could not see her body on the path. She then realised that she was actually inside the house, but emphasised that that was ok, because she was just about to put her running shoes on, get out of the armchair and turn the TV off. I asked her for the evidence. Was she about to put her shoes on etc.? She could not find any evidence that suggested she was planning to do any of these things.

Obstacles

What is in the way of achieving your goal?

Wisdom from the unconscious: The true advantage of working with the unconscious in art therapy will become obvious in this section and the next, which explores our strengths. We all have goals in life, but for various reasons some goals are extremely difficult to achieve, like in Jennifer's case of trying to lose weight. In her mind, she is pretty clear that she wants to lose weight, but for many years she has not been successful. She always went back to her old self-defeating eating habits and low-exercise regime. She felt jinxed. To set up another plan of dieting and exercise, felt like setting herself up for another failure. In her unconscious, however, there is an incredible wisdom that might help her after all. C.G. Jung talked about the collective unconscious, meaning that we participate in other people's unconscious through common experiences, memories and instincts inherited by our ancestors. This may seem a strange idea, and I believe many psychiatrists and psychologists thought the same in the early twentieth century, but if we look at current evidence in epigenetics, I can see a growing understanding of the way in which hereditary and historical patterns may emerge across generations. For more than a hundred years, people have been arguing whether we are more a result of nature or nurture, a result of biology or environment. But since the 1990s, with revolutionary synthesis in epigenetic change, we start to see influences that go both ways, e.g. how strong life experiences of our ancestors can affect our genes (Siegel, 2017) and how this goes back through many generations, very Jungian after all. Consequently, we not only have access in our unconscious to the wisdom from our own life, but we might also have access to the great positive and negative experiences of our ancestors. A true source of wisdom, which is unconscious to us, but might be visible in images.

When people draw goals, their unconscious often anticipates what is going to happen. If your unconscious does not believe that you can lose weight for example, it is probably going to show it in the picture, often in a cryptic way, or indicating your own obstacles, or sometimes bluntly showing that you are actually not doing what you think you are.

Looking at the picture

Now have a look at your own Goal Drawing and let's investigate what your obstacles might be. What your unconscious is trying to tell you that might be in the way of achieving your goal. An obstacle is not a bad thing. In actual fact, your unconscious is trying to assist you to achieve your goal, but presents the obstacles to show you what is in the way or what you are doing to create the obstacle. This is important information, so when your own obstacles appear in your Goal Drawing you need to face them. Your unconscious wants you to take the obstacles seriously so that you can change your life to reach your goal. I often find obstacles in the picture by looking for things that are not quite right; but remember that the client has to discover the obstacles for themselves.

Questions: please take notes

What obstructions to achieving your goal are in the picture? What is missing? This might be an obstacle. What are you facing? What are you not facing? Is there a section of your image that makes you feel uncomfortable, that did not work out the way you wanted? Is there a part of your drawing that you couldn't get quite right, that looks strange in a way? How could that be an obstacle to achieving your goal?

Back to case example: Jennifer's goal

Let's look at Jennifer's picture and try to hypothesise what her obstacles could be.

It showed her sitting in an armchair in the left-hand side of the picture and on the right hand side was a TV playing. In the middle of the picture, you could see a large window that showed the outside garden. There was a path in the garden leading into a forest and there was a little dog outside that was jumping up and down in front of the window.

I often have a hypothesis, but I don't assume anything as it might just be my projection, and the answer always needs to come from the client. So I asked her, 'What in the picture, could hold you back from running in the forest?' She said that nothing could hold her back. She noted that she was about to get up, turn the TV off and leave with her dog. I asked her to explain what she was doing in the picture and if that could possibly interfere with her plan? This is the moment when she noticed something and began to smile, like she was caught by her parents in the lolly shop with extra lollies in her pocket. In my experience, when the unconscious becomes conscious, clients often change their posture, or visibly show a change in their emotions. I asked her what she was thinking or feeling, ". . . right now". She said that the old patterned, leather armchair could stop her from going outside and exercising. I asked her to tell me more about it. She said that the armchair was given to her by her mother, and her mother got it from her mother. The armchair has since been her place of refuge, her safe place, a place to be when things were bad or when she needed some comfort, (a bit like Early Childhood Resources – see Chapter 2). She would often sit in the chair, having platters of food on her knees or on the little table next to her, while watching TV. I asked her what other thing in the room or in the picture could hold her back from getting up and putting on her running shoes. She indicated the TV, because she loves watching it and spent many hours every day in front of it, having only two days of work per week. It appeared to me that the armchair and the TV were her obstacles in losing weight. Most of us would think that this would be obvious to Jennifer, however it was a huge revelation seeing it in the picture.

Now that Jennifer is aware of her obstacles being obstructions to her goal, we can ask her to let go of worrying about how much time she spends on that couch, watching TV, and ask her to focus instead on her unique strength. In my opinion, our strengths are what help us reach our goals and not the focus on our obstacles.

Strengths

Our unconscious in all its wisdom does not want us to fail but to succeed. This is actually quite remarkable. People often get scared of unconscious ideas, impulses and perceived 'dark things' that are hidden within them. However, I have found that the unconscious is our friend. It shows us our dark sides and inner demons, but at the same time tries to indicate ways of overcoming our problems. This happens in the goal activity, when clients project unique strengths into their images, which can help them overcome their unique obstacles.

- Ask yourself now: What are your inner strengths that could help overcome your obstacles in achieving your goals? Please have a look at your picture and look for something strong or positive that might be able to help overcome the obstacles that you have found before, and write them down. The strengths will be in the picture.

- Is there an area of the picture you particularly like? An area that looks good, strong and convincing?
- How can this be a strength to overcome your unique obstacle?
- Can you visualise your strength?

Back to case example: Jennifer's goal

Let's examine Jennifer's picture again to find her strengths.

It showed her sitting in an armchair in the left-hand side of the picture and on the right hand side was a TV playing. In the middle of the picture, you could see a large window that showed the outside garden. There was a path in the garden leading into a forest and there was a little dog outside that was jumping up and down in front of the window.

I asked Jennifer, "What do you like in the picture, what could help you to get out of the armchair, turn the TV off, put on your runners, so you can go running?" Jennifer found two things that would do that for her. Number one was her **puppy**. I asked her about it, as I try not to assume anything. She told me that her puppy was her best friend and she loved him unconditionally and that he loved her. She would do anything for him. I asked her, "What does your puppy like the most?" This was an intuitive question. Trust your intuition, but don't assume you are right. She mentioned that her puppy likes running in the forest. I asked her if she takes him running regularly and she said, ". . . rarely", but when she does, they both really enjoyed it. I asked her what other aspect in the picture might be helpful to getting her out of the armchair and she mentioned the **forest**. She informed me that right behind her house there is a path that leads into this magical large forest and she loves exploring it for hours and running there with her dog.

Much of my thinking in working with the unconscious follows the principle **"Where attention goes, energy flows, where energy flows, life grows"**. Basically, if you focus on your strengths and not on your obstacles, then your goal is more likely to become a reality.

Summing up

- Summarise in two short sentences your own goals and your inner strengths that can overcome your obstacles in order to achieve it.
- Example: 'With this inner strength (name it), I'm going to overcome this obstacle (name it) to achieve my goal (name it)'.
- **Jennifer:** Focusing on my dog's needs and happiness, I am going to run with him into the forest as much as possible, so I don't worry any longer about sitting in my armchair or eating lots of food while watching TV.

Middle-term and long-term pictures

Please do the same exercise as above with your other two pictures and take detailed notes. Remember, doing these activities helps you to achieve your life goals, so they are worth every minute and every hour that you spend doing them.

Back to S.M.A.R.T

Now, this part gets very interesting. Remember the S.M.A.R.T. strategy, earlier in the chapter? If my clients had very troublesome problems or goals that were important but difficult to achieve, I found that the S.M.A.R.T. approach was never enough to make a real change. I imagine the S.M.A.R.T. approach works more for simpler or managerial problems and less for deep-seated psychological issues. However, in my experience as a psychologist, the S.M.A.R.T. approach actually works quite well when it is based on some prior work with the unconscious. Basically, we are doing cognitive-behaviour therapy after we have uncovered the depth of the issue.

Back to case example: Jennifer's goal

I suggested to Jennifer that we could set up a plan for her, so her goal to lose weight could be more concrete. We would look at what she would do and how she could achieve her goal. I asked her, "How often can you imagine going into the forest with your dog?" She told me that she used to go there every morning before breakfast and every evening before dinner. I asked her if that was still an option and she said that it should be easy as she only worked two days per week.

My behaviour modification for Jennifer using S.M.A.R.T.:

> I would like you to take your dog every morning before breakfast and dinner for a walk into the forest. I don't mind how long that is, as long you take him there. Don't worry about time, don't worry about sitting in your armchair, don't worry about how much TV you watch, and especially don't worry about what you eat at this stage. Just eat normally as you have done in the last few months without a conscious change of diet. We are shifting your focus to what your unconscious has suggested to you.

Follow-up with Jennifer: three years later

Living in a small community means that you can sometimes run into your previous clients, and when I ran into Jennifer, I was nicely surprised. Jennifer looked like she had lost half of her body weight, so I asked her about it. She informed me that she did exactly what we discussed, and the first couple of weeks she only went into the forest for about five minutes with her dog, but as time went by, she started to spend more and more time with him, exploring the native bushland and, ". . . got more and more lost in this magical space", chasing her dog around and finding beautiful objects. The previous year, she'd even made two new friends who continue to meet with her in the forest during the week, walking their dogs with her. She succeeded in losing weight, because she followed through on her insight into her strengths, giving more time to what she loved and therefore less time to eating in front of the TV. After a while, she felt less interested in junk food, and more like having healthier food, especially after a long walk.

Further notes on how to lead the therapeutic process

- **All the 'ah-ha' moments often come when we link the picture to the present.** This is crucial – it can help with the breakthrough. The aim is to get the client to open up. If they don't, they may be resisting. We try to bring them to the stage where they can connect. You can often see it in your client's body language. It's often about deep-seated fears. No one wants to look at what they are worried about. With art therapy you can get to what is relevant. If you encounter resistance, you can come back to it later. In my experience, if you really care about your clients, rather than confronting them too much, get them to slowly open up and they will have an insight when they are ready.
- **Respect the space of the client.** Make sure you don't push the client too strongly, especially if they show signs of resistance. Empower the client, so they can follow their own goals and achieve what they want to achieve. Don't take it personally if the client gets upset with you.
- **The process is more or less challenging.** As the therapist, it is important not to make judgements, and very important to give ownership of the process to the client.
- **Goal work is less structured**, more playful, exploratory and open minded, with a focus on the picture, themes, obstacles, and inner strengths. The future is less tangible, and we cannot be too structured about a vision in our mind, as we don't know how things will go.
- **Short-term goals** tend to be more pragmatic. **Medium-term goals** tend to be more emotional, about relationships or family focussed. **Long-term goals** are often dream-like in quality, playful and light; wishes awaiting fulfilment.

Additional tasks on goals

- Look at the three different pictures of your goals, the three different summary sentences that you have written. What are the commonalities? Focus on common obstacles and inner strengths. If some obstacles and strengths occur repeatedly, it might be a key obstacle or strength. Key strengths provide an easier focus, as you only have to focus on one thing to achieve several or all of your goals.
- If you feel inspired, look at the inner strengths and make a sketch, drawing or painting of that common inner strength, or the most important inner strength. This will support your new focus.

In my practice, I find that goal-based activities can be most beneficial towards the end of a counselling process. I particularly avoid using goal-directed activities with depressed clients at the beginning of therapy. This is due to the symptom of hopelessness that is normally part of the depressive experience and the difficulty depressed clients may have in forming positive ideas of their future. However, towards the end of treatment, especially with a depressed client, the art therapy goal activity can be a very productive and even fulfilling one. Children and young people with behavioural difficulties may also dislike goal work if they hold a negative outlook on their lives, if they are in trouble a lot, or if they receive messages from adults about how negative their future will be if they keep going the way they are. Towards the end of treatment, once things have changed to become more positive, these clients may also enjoy formulating and drawing up goals towards a brighter and more fulfilling future.

Literature

Siegel, D.J. (2017). *Mind: A journey to the heart of being human*. New York, London: Norton.

CHAPTER 6

Abstract art and the self-picture mind map

Elements of abstract art appear in many early cultures as signs or inscriptions on rocks, or marks and decoration on pottery, where simple geometric and linear forms were used. Form, colour, line, tone, and texture is found in all art, but in 1910 the painter Wassily Kandinsky, who described a true work of art as having emotional significance, where colour may dominate over form (Ehrich, 2011), portrayed his first nonrepresentational watercolour, which is considered the beginning of Abstract Art. Paul Cézanne is also considered one of the fathers of abstract art. He is credited for having influenced modern art movements, including Cubism, which rejected traditional art, especially perspective, and placed importance on emotional content.

Abstract art was at first confusing, even shocking, to the public as it did not represent the visible world and seemingly mocked the skill and artistic merit of realistic painters; however, the art movements of the early twentieth century were influenced by cultural change and most artists were searching for a new way to express their ideas and personal experience. Emotion and imagination were more important than how accurately the image depicted reality. Surrealism, with its emphasis on the unconscious and archetypal symbols, was influenced by ideas from Freud, Jung and Marx, and assisted the popularity of abstract art.

Abstract art allows expression of emotion and gives a sense of freedom to the artist, as there are 'no rules' in making the artwork look like anything real. Often, art therapists encourage their clients to do abstract images for that reason. The process and the arrising emotions become the main focus for later discussions.

In art therapy, the advantage of doing an abstract picture is that it puts no pressure on the client to draw or paint realistically as some clients will say they "can't draw". I often explain that like children we can draw straight or curved lines, shapes, forms, and use colours, which helps to counteract any standards of art a client might have. As being judgemental about the aesthetic end result is unnecessary for both the client and the therapist, I tell the client that the end result can look like anything, good or bad, beautiful or ugly, to help 'free them up' and explore their imagination, as what we are looking for is the essence, the emotional content, in the process. It's also quite intriguing how many clients also find that abstract art really frees them up, and they get a sense of how easy and fun it is to do this kind of art.

How do we read a clients abstract shapes, lines and colours?

Using 'art as therapy' and asking how the client felt while drawing the abstract images can lead to great insights. However, sometimes it can be a bit like fishing: you never know if the client will come up with something important that you can work with. This can be quite frustrating for clinicians, as most clients need urgent help and don't have the luxury to wait for several months or years for important ideas to emerge. I am not advocating for a quick fix here however, I am proposing an 'art in therapy' approach with abstract art, that might help practitioners to be more directive.

The result of the technique that I am using in this chapter is quite astounding as it allows a client to freely associate with their own abstract images, giving easier access to their unconscious, and helping them with insights they might not have had otherwise. 'Art in therapy' can be very therapeutic as the deeper meaning of shapes, colour, and movement in an abstract image is unveiled to the client.

Abstract self-picture: drawing task

Time: 1–2 hours

Materials: Acrylic, oil paint, or watercolours are best when working with abstract images, as the layering of colours is essential. In my sessions I find there isn't enough time between the drying of layers when using oil paint, so I give my clients 'Caran d'Ache Neocolor 1' oil crayons. I highly recommend a set of 15 or 30 crayons. They can be used to layer different levels of colour, one on top of each other, which normal oil crayons can't achieve. This gives the client an ability to 'paint' with crayons. They are expensive, but they last for a very long time.

Centre yourself first

You will need to centre yourself **and get in touch with yourself** before doing this drawing task. You might want to go for a walk first, find a park or some nature or do whatever you normally do to centre yourself before starting this picture, so that you can be calm and relaxed. "The self is not only the centre, but also the whole circumference [that] embraces both conscious and unconscious; it is the centre of this totality, just as the ego is the centre of consciousness" (Jung, 1971).

Close your eyes and feel the essence of who you are. Meditate for a couple of minutes in a non-judgmental way if possible.

- In which part or parts of your body do you experience/feel yourself most; where are you aware of being '*you*'?
- If you are Buddhist, you might believe that there is no permanent you. You might want to free yourself from the false perception, from the illusion of self,

but in this case we are talking in a Jungian sense of the self, the whole circumference of the conscious and unconscious mind, and those experiences that are positive and negative that have shaped you so far.

- Concentrate on an area of your body, where you experience yourself most, and sit with it for 2–15 minutes.
- Then open your eyes and create an abstract picture of yourself. Try to draw yourself with different colours and shapes without relying on concrete or figurative things in your environment such as houses and trees. Try to avoid symbols i.e. religious symbols, yin and yang, flowers or hearts, and written words. (It's acceptable if symbols emerge out of the abstract drawing or painting, but try to intentionally avoid symbols, so the deeper meaning can surface). Fill the entire page with colour. If you want to have something white, use a white crayon, but please don't leave any parts of the picture blank. Explore the details about yourself and spend at least one hour doing the abstract self-picture. Take time for this task and don't simplify it. Explore your inner self mindfully, with full awareness. Awareness of your emotions, your body and any part of yourself that you become conscious of.

Describe your self-picture

Take notes: How does the picture look? Collect qualities/metaphors for your picture without censorship and judgment.

You may have found a couple of descriptions, words, perhaps, even a nice metaphor, but you may also find that you are running out of ideas pretty quickly doing this by yourself. Ideally, you would have an art therapist sitting next to you who is prompting you to come up with descriptions and deeper associations.

Most art therapists seem to use abstract images more as 'art as therapy', as it can be quite difficult to know what to ask a client when looking at something abstract. In art therapy, and also counselling in general, you normally ask about the story, which is more evident in concrete and figurative pictures. In non-representational or abstract pictures, how do we enquire and prompt about something that has apparently no story, or seemingly nothing the client can just talk about? The leading question is, how do we do 'art in therapy' with abstract images?

Part of the answer lies in the mind's ability to try and define anything it sees. Our brain is constantly assessing what it sees and putting meaning into it. We are meaning makers (Kegan, 1982). Curtis (2011) sees shape, colour and content as the key aspects when viewing images. There have been others like Quail and Peavy (1994) who have used a similar list for viewing abstract images incorporating colour, spacing, pattern, texture, movement, tone and subjective images, or Betensky (1995) who understood forms, colour, movement and spacing as being the key aspects. None, however, appears to have used this list for 'art in therapy', exploring the unconscious material in the image. When I studied art therapy in Germany, I was introduced to an approach through the art therapists Otto Hanus, Birgit Naphausen and Maria Thomaser on how to use key aspects of abstract images for 'art in therapy'. Their understanding of these aspects greatly influenced this chapter. They focused on forms, colour, movement, and spacing. Of course, there are, and will be, ways of extending this list. At the moment, I am quite happy with using mainly four, although over the years my students have insisted we add another two aspects, which I have included later in this chapter.

A.   Describe the main aspects and explore their deeper meaning

1.   *Forms, shapes and lines*

Forms and shapes in abstract images can sometimes address aspects of your ability to structure yourself – the ability to create order in your life. Forms in abstract images can also reveal a lot about your 'soul', about the essence of 'you', with boundaries towards the world within (intrapsychic) and outside yourself (interpsychic). It may even indicate something about spirituality: 'to create a form', 'to be whole'. This is only a working hypothesis and we always have to check with our client as to how they interpret the images, allowing the client to describe, so that their projections can be uncovered. Nonetheless, this hypothesis can be very helpful, as it gives you some idea as to what 'forms and shapes' might be all about. For example, if a client has trouble creating a shape or form, they could have a problem with their sense of wholeness. Some clients struggle with boundaries towards others, and they often choose to create an outline of their form that is indistinct, or too thin, or a line with too many spaces in between. Some clients struggle with not being able to create close relationships, and their forms are sometimes rigid, the outlines too thick, perhaps with sharp edges and corners. Some clients have no sense of themselves or others and all their forms are just moving into each other without any boundaries or outlines.

How do you describe an abstract form and line?

They can be described as sharp, little, thin, large, stereotypical, whole, with thick armour, hollow, multi-layered, indistinct, deteriorating, cut off, string edge, soft, fragile, vulnerable, invasive, etc.

   As you ask your clients to describe the forms, shapes and lines in their abstract images, you will get a good sense of how they feel about themselves and others.

Forms, shapes and lines in your self-picture

Now have a look at your abstract image again, your 'self-picture'. Try to describe the forms, shapes and lines you see in the picture and add the descriptions to the list that you have started before. Furthermore, translate the picture qualities/ metaphors into psychological qualities if necessary. What psychological qualities can you see in your descriptions, the variables? For example, what does a thick line mean to you? Protected, armoured, rigid?

2. Colour

There is a great deal written about colour theory, the meaning of colours and how they impact on the viewer and how and why we use certain colours in art. But in 'art in therapy' colours in abstract images can be described according to how warm and cold they are, how strong or soft etc. Clients will often have many personal associations with specific colours, such as this colour looks bright, cool, dark, transparent, monochrome, it covers up, too bright, fragile, clear and strong, muddy, creates a strong contrast, has multiple layers, is diverse, harmonious, dissonant, rich, a poor choice, the list is endless.

Psychologically speaking, the colours we use in drawing often describe how we feel in the moment; our different emotions; our ability to express those feelings and recognise feelings in others. In my experience, if someone is able to express different feelings clearly, they are quite able to work with lots of colours in a differentiated and deeply felt way, rather than just using a few colours or just black and white in a 'tedious' and detached way. This does not mean that someone who draws mostly in black and white or uses very few colours in a simplistic way does not have feelings, but for most clients it might indicate that they may not be very skilful when talking about these feelings or picking up on the feelings of others. Colours are all about nuances of feelings, noticing them and being able to talk about them.

I have often wondered about great artists who have the ability to sense how different colours feel and work together, and if that might be a link to their own understanding of deeper feelings and more complex emotions. Although many great artists have been able to express their emotional sensitivity through magnificent colour in their artworks, it does not necessarily mean they were able to deal with their own emotions very well, as in the case of Van Gogh, who was considered rebellious and eccentric, and had many episodes of depression in his life. His brother, Theo, tried to persuade him to paint more like other artists in order to sell, but Vincent could not control his need for painting fast, and emotionally, with large amounts of paint on his brush, (Naifeh & White Smith, 2012) and with brilliant colours.

What does this knowledge about colours and emotions mean for art therapy?

It suggests there is a correlation between the way a person uses colour and their emotional intelligence. If you have a client, for example, who is very skilful with using colour, you might find that she can easily talk about her feelings and that she is able to pick up on the feelings of other people in her environment too. Alternatively, if you have a client who is very simplistic in her colour use, and prefers black and white, you might find that she is not very open to talking about her own feelings, is quite simplistic about them, and might also struggle sensing the feelings of other people. Both of these examples show a correlation between colour use and emotional intelligence. There are, of course, exceptions to the rule, as always when working with different types of individuals, and especially with the unconscious. I try not to follow any assumptions when working with clients, but it is interesting how often this correlation occurs.

Often, as art therapists, we might find ourselves having to do two jobs as we help our clients develop other aspects of themselves. We can use **art education** to teach our clients about the use of colour and artistic styles, and at the same time, do some **psycho education** where we teach them about feelings, help them to develop a language about feelings, how to recognise them, how to rate them and how to express them, etc. ('feeling picture cards' might be a good starter for this).

Colour in your self-picture

Have a look now at your abstract image again, your 'self-picture'. Try to describe the different colours you see in the picture and the way they make you feel and add the descriptions to your list, which you commenced earlier. Translate the picture qualities/metaphors into psychological qualities if necessary. What psychological qualities can you see in your descriptions? For example, what feeling does orange represent? It could be warm, cosy, embracing me like a thick and soft blanket on a winter morning. Be playful in your descriptions. There is no right or wrong. It is what it is for you. You own the meaning of your picture, nobody else does.

3. Movement and lines

We can often interpret and associate something to a shape or colour quite easily, but it might be harder to understand what movement means in abstract pictures. Frequently, an abstract picture will show lines, or shapes or colours that go in certain directions. This can happen with a straight or curvy line, or a back and forth line or a chaotic one, and there are many variables. Clients have been known to describe the movement in their pictures as rigid, stuck, controlled, explosive, rhythmic, calm, short, stopped, etc.

The psychological component of movement encompasses our emotions and flexibility. Movement in abstract images can be interpreted to represent the emotional state or change of the client, and the question "are you moved by what's going on in your life at the moment?" is a good starting point. Movement can sometimes depict strong feelings. For example, anger might be represented with a very sharp and direct brush stroke from one object to another one. Being emotionally overwhelmed might be represented with lots of lines in different directions, whereas feeling calm might be represented with very little movement and direction, or with a horizontal line or shape, or a round object. Feeling stuck might be represented with no movement options, or with a strongly enclosed shape, which may open up a discussion about lack of flexibility in someone's life.

Movement in your self-picture

Once again, have a look at your abstract image, your 'self-picture'. Try to describe the movement and its direction as you see it in the picture, as well as the way it makes you feel. Add descriptions to the list that you started before. Translate again the picture qualities/metaphors into psychological qualities if necessary. What psychological qualities can you see in your descriptions, the variables? For example, what does a lot of movement in your image stand for emotionally? Chaos, feeling stressed, freedom?

4. Space and relationship

The space and relationship aspect of the drawing or painting on paper or canvas is sometimes an indication of 'you' in relation to your 'space' in life and your 'relationship' to others and the world. The leading question is: Where are the objects, colours and movement located on this A4 or other format space and how do they relate to each other?

For example, abstract objects representing you and your mother, could be close, distant, on opposite ends, oppositional, overlapping and enmeshed, relating to each other or not, or moving towards each other. A good question would be, "How does that make you feel?" Objects can also be moving away from each other, or they can be similar, colourful or just different. One could ask, "How does that difference make you feel?" and other similar questions.

In psychological terms, the space aspect has to do with observational and relational skills. How do you relate to things and people in your environment, how are you orientated in your world? Space is about awareness of relationships within (intrapsychic) or outside of ourselves (interpsychic).

An art therapist might ask: Look at the space – how is it organised? Is it three-dimensional or two-dimensional? Are there different colours that relate to each other, or maybe it is organised at the bottom but not at the top? And how is that for you? Who or what is the orange shape in the middle, which is warm and centred? Who or what does it represent in your life? How does it relate to the dark black sharp edged shape at the top left corner? Who or what does that represent in your life, that is dark? What about the foreground, background, left, right, etc.?

Space in your self-picture

Looking at your abstract image again, your 'self-picture', try to describe the spatial aspects you see in the picture and add the descriptions to the list you have started before. How do the different objects, colours and perhaps movements relate to each other? How do they feel towards each other? Not all aspects are necessarily equally important. Some pictures are all about the shapes and others all about colour. Again, translate the pictures qualities/metaphors into psychological qualities if necessary. What psychological qualities can you see in your descriptions?

For example, what does the distance between you and the dark object stand for? Perhaps it's fear, resentment, frustration, or a great relief. For example, if your stepfather is too close to you in the image, how does that feel and how does this relate to your life experience with your real stepfather etc.

5.   Light

The next two aspects were suggested by my students. The aspect of light seems to relate mostly to the experience of light and darkness in one's life and when working with a client we need to be careful not to judge this as either good or bad. If I have learned anything in the last 25 years of working with the unconscious, it is to let go of my judgments. In psychology however, I was taught to build a hypothesis about what is going on for a client. This never sat well with me. I can see the point for the short term, but there is a great danger in projecting and generalising your interpretation onto the individual client. I believe it's better to listen well in a Rogerian and non-judgmental way. Investigate with your clients what these areas represent for them.

Light can be about how dark or light different areas appear, but also some colours are by nature more light than others. A frequent description with clients is 'contrast' when it comes to light and dark in an image, as it might refer to a contrast in their life. Psychologically speaking, lighter areas are often associated with positive experiences and darker areas with negative experiences. This might be linked to the experience of the daylight in comparison to the night where 'scary' and 'bad things' can happen. This is only a hypothesis however, and you will be surprised how many clients do associate dark areas with something positive, e.g. mysterious, deep, and meaningful. Therefore, allow the client to describe and interpret. Clients who describe the light and darkness in a picture might use words like bright, brilliant, polished, radiant, intense, dazzling, happy, light, friendly, scary, obscure, hidden, lost, forgotten, hiding, dingy, cave, murky, nebulous, pitch-black, vague, shaded, faint, light at the end of the tunnel, etc.

Light in your self-picture

Have a look at your abstract image again, your self-picture. Try to describe the light aspects you see in the picture if you have any, and add descriptions to your list that you started before. If this aspect doesn't apply to you, ignore it. Again, translate the picture qualities/metaphors into psychological qualities if you can. What psychological qualities can you see in your descriptions? For example, the white in the right top corner might represent space, freedom, lightness or a new life.

6.   Texture and sensual aspects

We can also investigate the texture and how it appears to our senses, especially touch. This is especially important when it comes to 3D objects like sculptures. This aspect probably doesn't apply to your abstract self-picture.

When clients describe their sculptures they might use words like smooth, soft, silky, delicate, comfy, vulnerable, rough, repulsive, jagged, spiked, thorny, sharp – "I am afraid of getting hurt by touching it", gooey and yucky, disgusting, sickening, creepy, strange and mysterious, unknown, formless, confronting, repugnant, etc.

Texture and sensual aspects of your self-picture

As you have done previously, you can apply descriptive words to your self-picture about the texture and sensual aspects if there are any.

B.   Mind mapping of the descriptions or themes

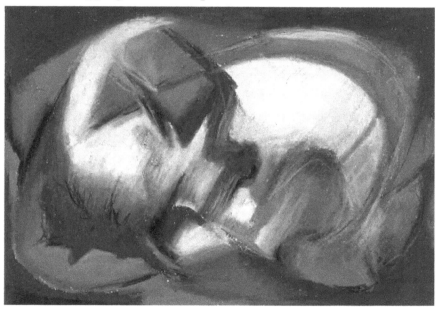

I came across mind mapping when I was studying psychology and realised what an important role it could play when working with abstract images.

The problem that sometimes occurs during this process is the client may give you too many descriptions in a chaotic order. Some are going to relate to forms and lines, some to colours and movements, and some to the space aspect, which may become overwhelming to manage. When working with figurative images, finding order is much easier. The client tells you a story and you can follow the client's thoughts by looking at the images and identifying, for example, who is walking on the beach, where they are going and what they are doing. But abstract images by their very nature are not identifiable, making it much harder to follow a client's description. The client tends to move around the drawing quite randomly without necessarily having a clear order in their mind.

As a therapist you may also struggle in following and 'getting the picture' of what is going on for the client. You may end up having lots of descriptions, but not knowing how they relate to each other and what they mean. Also, your client might struggle to relate and connect the descriptions with their own life as the unconscious content is likely to be 'all over the place,' and rather confusing. So, in this critical next step you will find it much easier to structure the information the client gives you by using mind mapping, creating order out of the chaos.

A mind map is like a geographical map, but instead of showing different countries, it shows the 'inner map' of a person, what is going on deep inside them, but in an ordered way. To create this 'inner map', you will need to listen carefully to the different descriptions your client provides and order them according to the main themes that come up. I normally find about three to five themes where everything seems to 'gel' together. If you have too many themes however, it might get chaotic again.

Mind map your self-picture

Now have a look at all your descriptions. This will take some time. Get another piece of paper or use your journal, and re-write all the words, but this time order them according to themes and topics that belong together. For example, you might have, 'the good yellow parts' of your picture, your 'dark scary shapes on the left side' and other themes that emerge. When I work with clients, I not only write down the word descriptions, but I start mind mapping straight away, as I investigate shapes, colours, movement and space. This will become much easier as you gain experience. I have given you an example with 'Melissa' of how this might work, further down in this chapter. You can have a quick look now, before attempting this task.

C.   Order your mind map

When you have different themes, you might not really know where to start and where to finish when reading these themes back and summarising this information to the client. Therefore, you need to decide on how the story, which connects the different themes, flows best and relates best to the clients current issues. This is where clinical experience comes in handy, but even a beginner can do this by following some practical steps. For example, I often start with the positive theme and finish with the current issue, but other times I might start with the problem the client has identified and bring it to a positive ending that becomes apparent in the picture. You kind of need to use your gut feeling to decide how the story flows. Mind mapping is like unfolding a story!

You might think that following your intuition does not sound very scientific and psychologists often tend to be very proud of their scientific evidence-based approach and reasoning. Neuroscientists have found, however, that there are neurons in our gut. Just google Dan Siegel, neuroscience, and gut feeling. Therefore, even as a therapist, following your gut feeling is a valid approach and might help enormously as a strategy in art therapy.

Finally, you could give the themes an order with numbers, so an interesting story might emerge with a clear start, main themes and an ending. Number one for the start of the story and the last number for the end of the story, the last theme. This will help you to keep track of the different themes.

Order your self-picture

Now it's your turn to give order to your self-picture mind map. Make a choice about what comes first, next and where you want to finish. Sometimes, I just go with the order that the clients have used when they described their images but if you are doing this yourself then choose an order that feels right.

D.   Relating the story to the client's life and their current issues

In the next step, you read the story back to the client without referring to the pictures any longer, but focusing all the descriptions in order to relate to the client's current life and issues. As you read the story back to the client, you can check in with them; ask how this or that relates to his or her life at the moment; (abstract images are phenomenological, i.e. they are about the here and now). This process of 'art in therapy', where you write down the descriptions and read them back, relating them to the client in context to their life, is when the 'aha moment' often happens.

Relating the story back to your self-picture

If you have a friend or partner for this section who can read the story back to you and can 'play' the art therapist, you might find it easier to visualise how it relates to your life at the moment.

Example: chaotic

The theme might be chaotic, messy and all over the place.

Art therapist: Your life appears to be quite chaotic and messy at the moment, with many aspects of your life being all over the place, and I am wondering if you could tell me something about it? Where do you experience chaos in your life at the moment and how do you deal with it? Can you give me an example?

When you are relating the descriptions, reading them in order back to the client, it often feels to them that you are a bit like a clairvoyant, as they cannot imagine how you would know all this information about them. Often, clients forget what they have said about their pictures. By hearing your 'interpretation', they connect with something deep inside and forget what they have said before about their artwork.

Example: self-picture of a client

I have not included her picture here for confidentiality reasons.

Melissa initially described the colour in her self-picture as "mainly soft, open and flowing". I mind mapped this description and many others, ordered them and then asked her if she could relate to the idea that there is 'a softness' in her life, where she feels 'open' and 'things are flowing'.

She told me about the recent changes in her life, the new friendships she had made, the job where she could help the elderly and how she felt very 'soft' towards everyone. She also mentioned the openness that she always had, but also how the art therapy got things 'flowing' for her.

Melissa said that a separated, closed section in her picture looked like a "lock down", where the shapes were "really rigid and set", and this section was "dark and scary". I asked her, "What in your life feels like a 'lock down', where things are 'rigid and set'?" She told me about her husband's addiction and how she tries to separate this aspect from the rest of her life, but sometimes feels the "lock down takes over everything". I asked her if that was visible in the picture, that the "lock down takes over everything". She described how the closed section seems to be moving towards the soft centre. I asked her how that feels, and she said, "overwhelming, extremely scary", and that she can sense, "a great fear of losing everything".

When questioned, she said she felt "overwhelmed about my husband's addiction, extremely scared", and has a "great fear of losing everything" (the next theme). She started crying, and informed me that she had no idea how great her fear really was, and that she kept pretending that everything was okay. As long as she was helping others, she could keep ignoring the addiction and be nice to everyone. Secretly, she understood now that she had been lying to herself all along, and she realised she could not keep that part of her life out any longer for she knew something needed to be done.

As one of the key elements of abstract art is emotion, it lends iself well to art therapy, where even if you think you are just making stuff up, choosing colours randomly or just expressing yourself openly, the emotional content of your unconscious is so connected to communicating that which is most important to you, in colour, shape and lines that you will be able to reflect what is truly going on in yourself, on a deep emotional level, and insights will be gained. Perhaps this is why modern artists like Van Gogh, Picasso, and Pollock moved away from realism where one consciously works to make the picture resemble something in reality, but by using abstract art they could bring their emotional life, themselves, their own story into the picture, allowing their unconscious to express itself freely.

Literature

Betensky, M. (1995). *What do you see? Phenomenology of therapeutic art expression*. London: Jessica Kingsley Publishers.

Curtis, E.K. (2011). Understanding client imagery in art therapy. *Journal of clinical art therapy 1*(1), 10.

Ehrich , J (2011). *Zen art: Origins in abstract expressionism and art therapy.* Half Moon Bay: Zenjo Press.

Jung, C.G. (1971). *The portable Jung.* New York: Viking.

Kegan, R (1982). *The evolving self: Problem and process in human development.* Cambridge: Harvard University Press.

Naifeh, S., White Smith, G. (2012) *Van Gogh: The life.* London: Profile Books.

Quail, J., & Peavy, V. (1994). A phenomenologic research study of a client's experience in art therapy. *The Arts in Psychology 21*(1), 44–49.

CHAPTER 7

Self-Box: Become authentic and integrate traumatic memories

Trauma comes from the Greek word 'wound'. We normally think of trauma as a psychological wound, but the body is affected as well.

Being exposed to trauma, especially from abusive relationships, is a vital cause of many conditions effecting people's mental, physical and emotional well-being (Herman, 2015). Many practitioners and researchers have found that the trauma experience sits in the area of the brain that is also responsible for sensory and visual information. "Traumatic memories lack verbal narrative and context and are encoded in the form of vivid sensations and images" (Herman, 2015, p. 38). Neuroimaging studies show that traumatic experiences deactivate the left frontal cortex, particularly the Broca's area, which is responsible for speech (Talwar, 2007). It appears that the trauma experience is not entirely cognitive, but is a sensory one as well. The body is locked into a terror state and the horrors can't be articulated (Levine, 2010; Rothschild, 2000). The individual may have pushed the trauma behind a 'wall' to avoid the distress (Greenwald, 2009); however, the memory of the traumatic experience can resurface at any time. The trauma has a physiological basis, and the symptoms have their origin in the entire body's response to the original trauma (Van der Kolk, 2014).

Art therapy has been found to make a unique contribution to the process of recovery. As the trauma is locked in the visual area of the brain, expressing the experience visually is often not difficult for clients. While they are creatively expressing their inner terrors, externalising them on paper, they seem to start processing them, pulling them out of their non-verbal memory banks, (implicit), into verbal memory (explicit). Once the brain makes sense of it all, it appears that the body can let go of the trauma. Subsequently, talking therapy can have a place.

An art therapist may use simple drawing exercises to help a client tune into what is happening in their body and begin to identify their feelings. Asking "What does that colour mean to you?", and other questions to help guide the client. A great technique for trauma work is the rosebush strategy from the American Gestalt therapist Violet Oaklander (1997). While drawing a rosebush, clients can express the thorns in their lives, the lack of nurture and many things for which they might not have found words. This activity might remind the reader of the tree picture we discussed earlier, where trauma is sometimes expressed by showing extreme damage to the tree.

The Self-Box technique

Theory

I have found the *Self-Box* or Jungian box to be one of the most popular art therapy techniques in the world. The box, often an empty shoe box, is painted and decorated with different materials that symbolise '*You*'. The American psychologist and art therapist Margaret Naumburg seems to have originated this technique in the 1940s based on Jungian theory. The point of the Self-Box technique is to understand our inner and outer self, and to create a balance on how we reveal or conceal ourselves to others. The technique can help us creatively integrate the inner and outer parts of ourselves, if these are unbalanced. I have found the Self-Box to work particularly well with many kinds of issues, including clients who have experienced deep trauma.

Outside the box, shows how we represent ourselves to the world to impress others and/or how we avoid getting hurt; it is the superficial self. C. G. Jung talked about the '*persona*' in this context. The word '*persona*' is a Latin word meaning 'mask' or false face, and this was a theatrical mask used by Roman actors through which they spoke. Our persona or mask can sometimes be very powerful and provides a way to role-play aspects of ourselves, and also allows us to hide who we really are. In this way, the persona is a form of self-protection and can be useful at times. For example, in social situations when anxiety occurs, and we feel vulnerable, we may use our persona to protect ourselves. The negative trade-off is that we might get used to presenting a false facade and even start to forget who we truly are. The moment we want to create closeness to others, our mask will be in the way.

Fritz Perls (Gestalt therapy) believed that we need to unfold the client's personality so they can become more authentic. A bit like peeling an onion, where the first layer is the phony or cliché layer, which represents the games we play and the roles we get lost in (Perls, Hefferline, & Goodman, 1951).

One question to ask our clients and ourselves is, '*Do we want to keep the mask on the entire time, keep playing those games, keeping others at arm's length, and never experiencing closeness or intimacy?*'

Inside the box, shows what is creative in us and vulnerable. It represents our wants and needs, our emotional pain and personal life experiences. Inside is the real 'you'; no mask, just the 'intimate you'. Can we allow ourselves to be real? We all have insecurities and often overcompensate for them. However, when we are honest, and let go of our mask, we have an opportunity to deeply connect and become wise and compassionate.

Task: making the Self-Box

Time: Allow 2–4 hours for this activity.

Materials: Shoe box, scissors, glue, sticky tape, plain or coloured paper, paints and brushes, soft or oil crayons, egg carton containers (for mixing the paint), other materials of your choice such as pipe cleaners, paddle pop sticks, cotton wool, leaves, branches, rocks, cones, shells, glittery things like jewellery, 'bling', shiny-looking objects, anything you find around you and in nature, etc. Choose any materials and colours you want to express who you are from the inside and the way others see you on the outside.

Instructions: Select a shoe box and start painting/colouring/collaging the **inside first**, without using words or writing – just drawing, painting and collage. Show who you truly are in a creative way, by using any materials you have gathered. You can do this figuratively or in an abstract way or a mixture of both.

Note: Words are great to use in art therapy, however images speak louder than words. If you use them in the Self-Box, there is a danger that you won't express yourself from the unconscious, but you may represent a conscious thought or idea instead. The moment you are using colours and materials, your unconscious will project regard-less of your conscious intentions. We cannot hide our true self behind our pictures, but we can hide more easily behind words.

Inside the box, show with colours and materials:

Express your real self, including what you don't show to others around you. Show what you tend to hide and hold inside. It may be deep emotions and feelings relating to great, important or even traumatic experiences. What is the 'real you' like? Don't be shy at this stage and try to be as honest as you can. You don't have to share this with anyone if you don't want to.

Outside of the box, show with colours and materials:

As you have expressed the inside of the Self-Box, you don't have to worry about who you really are, for now you can focus on how others see or perceive you. How do you present yourself to others and to the world around you? Don't use words and writing; instead, use drawing, painting or collage with the materials of your choice. How do you show or present yourself to others? How do you avoid being hurt (again)? How do you protect yourself? Do you tend to have a specific mask that people normally see, or do you wear different masks with different people?

Transition between inside and outside:

Is there any connection between the outside and the inside of the box? Do you have doors or windows or other ways of connecting them? How large or small are they, how open or closed, or protected are they? How might you share your private thoughts, feelings and experiences with people you want to be with or get close to? Some things may only be visible for some, and other things may be visible to everyone.

Note: I've had clients who have forgotten to put a lid on their Self-Box and others who've used a thick tight rope that they've spun around the box hundreds of times. Where do you see yourself?

Questions for personal reflection

If you do this activity with a client, I recommend starting the exploration from the outside, the opposite to the sequence in which it was created. This allows the client to slowly open up and feel safe. This is making the process more organic, especially since you are getting to know the client and physically seeing them from 'the outside'.

Outside

Please use your journal and take notes, as it helps to deepen your understanding.

What was the process like? Write it down in detail. While you were making the Self-Box, did you get very emotional at a certain point? What were you thinking and what part of the box were you creating at the time? How does it relate to your life? How would you describe the outside of your Self-Box? Come up with as many associations and metaphors as you can. This can relate to the representational features of the box but also to the abstract aspects, like shapes, colour, movement and space. What makes the box interesting? What makes the box boring? How would others describe it? How does the outside of the box protect you from getting hurt? How does it keep people away from you? Do you have any idea about what you might be protecting? How do you keep others away from what you are protecting, normally?

Let's look at the transition

How do you move from the outside to the inside of your Self-Box? Are there any doors or windows or other forms of access? What do they look like? Please describe them in detail. How do they feel? Freely associate the different feelings that come up with the different features and their descriptions. What area/s inside can be seen through the access points, if you have any? How does that feel?

Note: When working with a client, please be aware that when the lid comes off the box, the client may feel quite exposed and vulnerable. Therefore, be extremely careful and respectful here, and allow the client to take the lead. This is consistent with the general notions of art therapy working to externalise feelings into a safe container and allowing a person's inner world to be seen (Case & Dalley, 2014).

Inside

What is it like to take the lid off the box and expose who you are? What relationship is there between the outside and the inside of the box? Is the inside similar or different to the outside?

Note: The greater the difference of the inside to the outside, the more we can assume that the client has a strong reason to hide the true self. This façade, however, is in the way of creating real closeness in life.

Further questions

Describe now what is different in great detail. Where do you most see yourself inside the box? What else do you see inside the box? Familiarise yourself with your safe place. What part of the Self-Box do you like most? Choose one particular area.

What part of the Self-Box don't you like? It might be a part that did not work out in the making of the box, or it may look negative or even scary or awful to you. Choose one area only (remember this area for later). If the different parts in the box could talk to you, what would they say?

Reflections

Working with the Self-Box is deeply personal and can be very confronting

Through the Self-Box exercise, the true self is encouraged to come out, which can be very revealing and intimidating. There may be tears. All the pain and hurt of the past is still buried in our unconscious. It's often visible in the box, a great advantage of art therapy vs talking therapy, for the conscious mind is not aware of all that is in our unconscious. Also, our unconscious does not understand time like we do consciously. There is no future, past and present. It is all you, and the world around you, and whatever happened in the past can have a very powerful impact in the present. Many clients report that this confrontation feels like it has the same intensity in the present even though it happened so long ago. It is strongly believed that keeping such phenomena unconscious, trying to forget what happened, requires much more energy and time than dealing with them consciously and honestly; therefore liberating us from complex tasks and allowing us to live realistically, productively and joyfully (McWilliams, 2011).

The box is a process

Heraclitus, the Greek philosopher noted that, "Change is the only constant in life, and no man ever steps into the same river twice". Similarly, the Buddha believed that life is a river that continuously changes. Nothing is fixed and permanent. Actually, there is a strong belief that the more you allow change and impermanence in your life, the more you grow as a person.

Note: You could do two Self-Boxes in the course of therapy and see how things have changed and integrated. Art therapy has also been widely used for children who have experienced natural disasters and catastrophic events. Children who lived through Hurricane Katrina drew similar pictures of flooded cellars for months after the event. Malchiodi (2007) observed that children who have experienced trauma, in any form, will repeat the image until relief is found. She believed that not only the sensory aspects of the hurricane were able to be communicated but that the repetition provided a means of self-soothing and stress reduction.

1. Therapeutic goal of the Self-Box: get to know yourself better, become more authentic and find opportunities to become who you want to be

For this part of the process the client makes changes to the Self-Box to create a balance between the inner and the outer. The questions need to reflect previous answers. Some examples are given below.

Can you see the difference between the inside and outside of your Self-Box? What can you do to change the outside so it can be more like the inside? Visualise it first and then do it. Please keep taking notes as you start changing your Self-Box. If the outside, for example, is too chaotic, too neat, too . . ., then, look at the inside. What elements from the inside needs to be incorporated into the outside to make it work better? What do you want to bring out physically, artistically? What is private, what needs to stay there? What will people say if that comes out? Who will be shocked? Who do you want to let in? What can come out in a meaningful way? Change your outside slowly, carefully and gradually in a mindful, authentic way. This way it will give you positive feedback from others, if that is what you are after. Choose the right environment for things to change. It is not about provoking or hurting others. It is about becoming more and more your true self. Have a look at what materials or ideas you want from the inside to be on the outside and get new materials or paint to do that. See what emerges in your artwork and live this full-heartedly in your life.

Note: My clients often report that after they have changed their Self-Box, their life has started to change accordingly. As an art therapist, you can keep working on changes of the Self-Box and other complementary activities for many sessions. Art therapy is rarely a one-off event.

What about clients who don't have facades?

I have used the Self-Box technique with many clients over the last 25 years, and occasionally I've had a client who seemed to have no facades, where the lid of their box was missing and where the inside was very similar to the outside. Quite often, these clients would wear their heart on their sleeve. At first, I thought that these clients were in a perfect state of being, seemingly totally authentic. In the early 90s however, I stumbled upon an article in developmental psychology, where the author proposed that honesty isn't always good and claimed that lying, or being fake, can be a good survival strategy. So I started to question my extremely genuine clients, and found that some of them had actually suffered from experiences where people used and abused their openness. Some of them experienced forms of domestic violence and severe abuse, where they were not able to protect themselves. Finally, I came to think that these clients might just need the opposite of having a goal in this technique. Instead of helping them to become more genuine, I facilitated a process where they would create a lid for their Self-Box, a persona that is powerful enough to keep abusers at a distance. This experience with the Self-Box was so insightful that it led to some further knowledge. Clients who have gone through intense abuse or any form of trauma, often represented something negative on the inside of their Self-Box, which led me to the second goal.

2. Therapeutic goal of the Self-Box: integrate traumatic memories and negative experiences

What areas inside your Self-Box don't you like? What areas look like they are done badly or didn't work out, or feel negative in some way? If you were a chess piece and had to position yourself somewhere on the inside of your box, which area do you like least, and where would you not like to be? Describe this area in detail and take notes. Write down your descriptions, by looking at the colours, shapes and themes in this area and how they feel to you.

What area inside your Self-Box do you really like? What is your favourite area that is very different to the other area you have just described? If you were a chess piece, where would you like to place yourself? Describe this area, as you did before and take notes. What colours do you see? What do the colours look like and how do they feel? What shapes do you see? What do they look like and how do you feel about them? What themes are there and how do you feel about them?

Now, think of how you could minimise the negative area with the help of the positive area inside your Self-Box. You are not allowed to remove the negative area or to totally cover it with art materials, but you can connect the areas creatively with different materials, so that the negative area feels less negative. Often, my clients create a path between the areas and bring new elements, like the ones from the positive area into the negative area without changing the look of the positive area. For example, if the positive area has a lot of flowers, they might place flowers all the way towards and into the negative area.

Siegel (2001) argued that during early childhood development, the right part of the brain develops faster – the part that is responsible for emotions, etc. Then around the age of three, our left, verbal part of the brain becomes dominant. When people are traumatised, they often can't talk about their experience (Tinnin & Gantt, 2014). It appears to be locked inside their right brain hemisphere, where implicit memory exists, (but not explicit for this experience), the part that is not available for language. In my experience, images like the Self-Box, however, can access that part of our brain and facilitate integration, sometimes not verbalised at all, but then clients can start to find words when they see what they have been doing.

The actual drawing or creative expression of the trauma is a sensory motor exercise, so the feelings associated with the trauma are activated and released. The motor functions involved in art making and the focussed 'working' of an issue by physically creating it as an image or sculpture can aid the healing process (Lusebrink, 2010).

I would highly recommend you do this process, especially if you identify a negative area in your Self-Box that needs integrating.

Reflect

Look at the negative, dark, or painful area – has it changed? Does it feel less negative? How does it look and feel now? Describe and write down the changes.

We can learn to adjust to negative experiences. We can embrace the negative area of the Self-Box as described above, and emerge as a stronger, wiser and more compassionate person. Dan Siegel (2017, p. 79) summarised integration as being more "connected, open, harmonious, emergent, receptive, engaged, noetic (a sense of knowing), compassionate, and empathic". If integration is not achieved, he found that people often ended up in extremes of behaviour, either chaotic or rigid, as evident with most mental health disorders. I believe this might be a guide for clinicians asking themselves at the end of therapy, "Has my client moved on the scale between chaos and rigidity to the integrated and balanced centre or is more work still needed?"

If we suppress things, they can dominate our lives (like the Jungian 'shadow'). If we face it, we can move on and find our balanced and integrated centre. The darkness and 'shadow' in our life exists as part of our unconscious mind. It is composed of repressed ideas and experiences, inferior and guilt-laden personality traits, weaknesses, desires, instincts and shortcomings. This archetype is often described as the darker side of the psyche. The challenge in art therapy remains to assist our clients in facing their inner demons, gradually, in a safe environment that allows integration, rather than letting them continue to supress them, in an endless fight or flight.

Story of St George

Having worked with traumatised clients over many years, the image of St George often comes to mind. He was a Roman soldier and in Medieval times was often portrayed as a knight on the back of a white horse who would spear a dragon, the symbol of the demon. As a psychodynamic therapist, I've worked with clients who try to suppress uncomfortable and highly threatening experiences, i.e. the desire to kill this inner demon, and I've considered how deeply ingrained it is in their unconscious. As the stories tell us, once a dragon slayer has killed his prey, he can only abstain from killing for a while. By his nature, he keeps looking for further dragons to kill. Similarly, people try to kill their inner demon repeatedly and all their attention goes into it. Consider, 'Where attention goes, energy flows, were energy flows, life grows' (Huna Principle). So, the dragon, the inner demon, becomes bigger and bigger. With all the attention we give to our negative past, the demon always seems to 'pop' up when it is least wanted. An example of this suppression would be when we want to trust a new stranger in our life, but behave very anxiously.

I have seen a picture of St George in a German church where he did not kill the dragon, but instead put a necklace around his neck, which was attached to a metal chain that he was holding firmly in his hand. Now, this image represents true integration for me. When I have clients who emerge out of their work with their Self-Box truly integrated as a stronger and wiser person, they feel much more empowered. It's as if they have a dragon pet next to them; tame and quiet, but ready to strike when needed. This has become the aim of Self-Box work for me, assisting clients to face their inner demon, 'be-friend' the demon in a strange sort of way, where the clients learn to put their story and stressful experiences in a safe place, so that it no longer interferes negatively in their lives, or at least requires less attention, so they can move forward. Furthermore, I believe trauma results in broken trust and the treatment is about exposure, integration and learning to trust again. In this way, art therapy transforms "shit into gold", as one of my clients put it eloquently. Jung often depicted the therapeutic process as alchemy.

Case example, Self-Box, goal 1: Steph

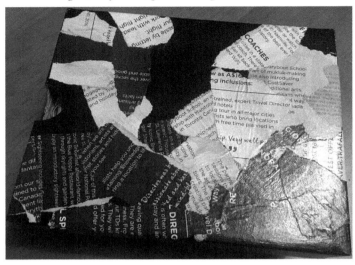

Rob: How does your Self-Box look on the outside?

Steph: It looks uneven, odd, dark and rough. It reminds me of Buffy the Vampire Slayer.

Rob: Do you present yourself a bit odd, perhaps even dark and rough like a vampire slayer when you want to keep others at arm's distance, so they don't get close to you?

Steph: I definitely didn't think about this when I made the box, but you are absolutely right. I can be quite odd and aggressive when I don't like somebody.

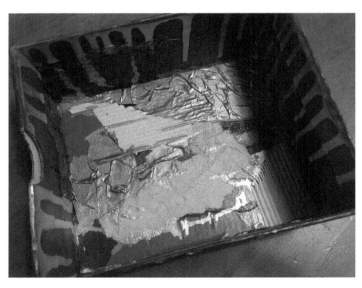

Rob:	How does the inside look different to the outside?
Steph:	It looks bright and shiny. It looks precious and special.
Rob:	What is your favourite part?
Steph:	I love all the gold and how it spreads.
Rob:	Is there anything on the inside that you could bring outside, that would more fully represent who you truly are?
Steph:	I would like to be more genuine with people I care for, so I can imagine having some golden spots on the sides, but not on the lid where everyone can see it.

Steph went home and did that.

Case example, Self-Box, goal 2: Helena

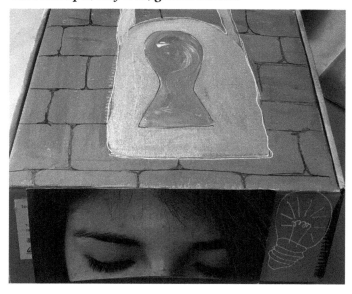

Rob:	Tell me about the outside of your Self-Box.
Helena:	It looks like a brick wall. It is not open for anyone. You can't go in, but you wonder what is inside. You can see the keyhole.
Rob:	What does the brick wall look like to you and how does it feel?
Helena:	It looks very organised, well maintained and there is a warmth to it.
Rob:	Do you present yourself to others as well organised and well maintained with some warmth?
Helena:	Yes, very much so. I like being organised and everyone knows that about me and I like looking after my appearance. I imagine some people perceive me as warm and caring.
Rob:	You mentioned that you are not open, more like a brick wall, but people wonder what is inside of you when looking at the keyhole.

Helena: I don't easily share personal stuff. I actually keep most things to myself, even with people I love. But I am also aware that people are quite curious to learn more about me, and I like their interest.

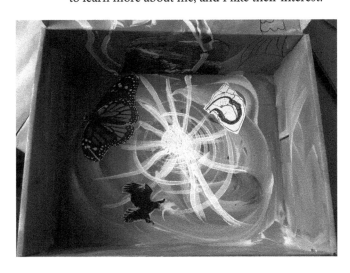

Rob: When you are looking inside your Self-Box, what comes to mind that is quite different?
Helena: The radiating sun in the middle that goes into different areas. I can feel a strength and joy there. I also like the flow of colours.
Rob: How is the flow of colours?
Helena: It is warm and energising, a bit like the sun in the centre.

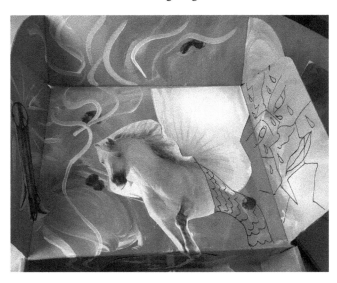

Rob: You have also added another layer to the inside that can be unfolded. What do you see there that you haven't mentioned yet?

Helena: I can see sadness and disappointment. I can see a face with a tear that is broken. I can see an outline that has no colour, but is just black.

Rob: Is there anything in your life now or has there been a time when you felt a strong disappointment that left you deeply broken and sad?

Helena: I know exactly what that was.

Rob: You can share this experience, but you don't have to. We can still work with it in a way that will make you feel better without having to talk about it.

Helena: I have talked about it for many years, and I don't want to tell the story any more, but I would love to change my feelings toward it.

Note: There is a great risk in psychotherapy in re-traumatising clients who don't want to talk about what happened, so we need to learn to be extremely perceptive and respectful of their wishes rather than following our own curiosity or the brief of family members or others. However, art therapy allows us to work on integration during the process, without having to talk about it; how great is that?

Rob: OK. Please tell me now, when looking at your Self-Box, what is your favourite area? Is there an area that can oppose the sad and broken area of your Self-Box?

Helena: I think it is the sun in the middle, but also the white horse that comes to mind. They are white, bright, light like a feather. I think of innocence and transformation through the spirit.

Rob: Is there a way you could connect those two areas, the broken sad one with the sun and the horse, so the broken sad area feels less broken, less sad?

Helena: Yes, I could paint a white line that goes through them and into the sad area. I could also add some colours to the face with the white lines.

Rob: Please do that when you go home today and bring the changed box back to our next appointment.

When she returned to our next session, she described the broken face as "less sad" and her disappointment had changed into acceptance. She also mentioned that the face looked "alive" and "warmer", and she could accept what had happened a bit better, and even forgive, a little more. Even though we never discussed her sad experience she certainly expressed that she was "less sad" about it through doing the Self-Box.

I hope these two examples have given you some ideas on how to work with Self-Boxes. I am not really following a therapeutic script as such, and the questions I've listed are an example of the possibilities. I try to go along with whatever the client brings up and keep my personal projections at a minimum. This becomes easier the more experience you have and the more you know yourself.

Literature

Case, C. & Dalley, T. (2014). *The handbook of art therapy* (3rd ed.). London, New York: Routledge, Taylor & Francis Group.
Greenwald, R. (2009). *Treating problem behaviours: A trauma-informed approach.* New York: Routledge, Taylor & Francis Group.
Herman, J.L. (2015). *Trauma and recovery: The aftermath of violence – from domestic abuse to political terror.* New York: Basic Books.
Levine, P. (2010, April). Interview by V. Yalom and M.H. Yalom with P. Levine: Peter Levine on somatic experiencing. Retrieved 27 June 2018 from www.psychotherapy.net/interview/interview-peter-levine
Lusebrink, V. B. (2010). Assessment and therapeutic application of the expressive therapies continuum: Implications for brain structures and functions. *Journal of the American Art Therapy Association 27*(4), 168–177.
Malchiodi, C. (2007). *The art therapy sourcebook* (2nd ed). New York: McGraw-Hill.
McWilliams, N. (2011). *Psychoanalytic diagnosis: Understanding personality structure in the clinical process* (2nd ed.). New York: Guilford Publications.
Oaklander, V. (1997). The therapeutic process with children and adolescents. *Gestalt Review 1*(4), 292–317.
Perls, F., Hefferline, R., & Goodman, P. (1951). *Gestalt therapy: Excitement and growth in the human personality.* London: Souvenir.
Rothschild, B. (2000). *The body remembers: The psychophysiology of trauma and trauma treatment.* New York: WW Norton.
Siegel, D. J. (2001). Toward an interpersonal neurobiology of the developing mind: Attachment relationships, 'mindsight', and neural integration. *Infant Mental Health Journal 22*(1–2), 67–94.
Siegel, D.J. (2017). *Mind: A journey to the heart of being human.* New York, London: Norton.
Talwar, S. (2007). Accessing traumatic memory through art making: An art therapy trauma protocol (ATTP). *The Arts in Psychotherapy 34*, 22–35.
Tinnin, L. & Gantt, L. (2014). *The instinctual trauma response and dual brain dynamics.* Morgantown: Gargoyle Press.
Van der Kolk, B. (2014). *The body keeps the score: Brain, mind, and body, in the healing of trauma.* New York: Viking–Penguin Books.

CHAPTER **8**

Creative Mind Ordering (CMO):
Change neural pathways

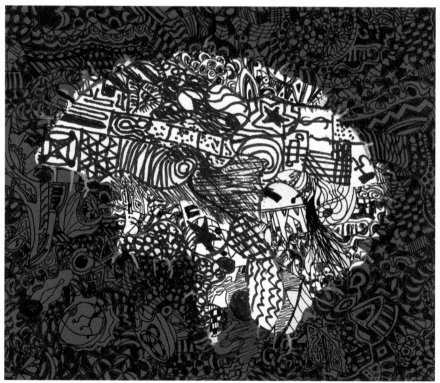

Dean Bridle, 2017

Art therapy has always had an art-based philosophy integrated into its practice, where creativity and personal experience have played a role. Therefore, this style of therapy has encountered resistance to being compatible with scientific principles. However, since the advancement of neuroscience, a field that has highly contributed to research of brain activity, recent studies have been able to evaluate some of the effects of art therapy on different brain regions, showing how the brain and body respond to art related experiences.

Neuroscience has come a long way in understanding the human brain, as not so long ago it was believed that the brain did not grow past adulthood. Today, however, it is very well established that the brain grows, i.e. continues to produce new cells, throughout our lifespan (Siegel, 2017). Through brain scans, neuroscience can help scholars further investigate the neurological activity in the brain and therefore create links between neurological and psychological states.

As more research is conducted on emotional states, stress levels and the nervous system, art therapy is gradually being supported by scientific data. Among practices like meditation and yoga, which have been operating in global cultures for thousands of years, art therapy has become of interest to many researchers of 'mind–body medicines' or psychoneuroimmunology. Researchers propose, since stress may increase the probability of diseases, that a more holistic approach to healing is of great benefit to patients (Lorenz, 2006).

Art therapy can successfully enhance neurogenesis, creating new connections in the brain, to resume functioning of injured brains through intensive and sustained rehabilitation (Chia-Shu et al., 2013). It can help in the treatment of traumatic brain injury, TBI, with a focus on cognitive issues, improving memory and the attention span (Malchiodi, 2013).

Images can be a bridge between body and mind, or between the conscious levels of information processing and the physiological changes. Neuroscience research shows that imagery we see, or we imagine, activates the visual cortex of the brain in similar ways. In other words, our bodies respond to mental images as if they are reality (Malchiodi, 2012). Through art therapy interventions and the continued use of positive and useful neural pathways of thinking, it is possible to change emotional and destructive behavioural patterns.

Creative Mind Ordering (CMO)

If we were robots, we could have an inbuilt switch we could turn on and off for our emotions so that whenever something bad happened we could use the switch to turn off the anger or sadness. Being human, our brains are wired to respond, sometimes so quickly without thinking, that when it happens, we might not be able to control our emotions.

The following is the most complicated approach in art therapy I have ever come across; however, it allows us to look at how our thinking occurs when we respond and it attempts to change neural pathways through uncovering an unconscious inner strength. Neurological pathways are created and developed at an early age in response to an event or repeated events that we call the 'trigger'. When the event is distressing or inhibits personal growth, a symptom, in the form of an unpleasant, painful or negative thought or feeling, develops. When that event is continually repeated or is particularly traumatic then the pathway strengthens, and the symptom is easily *triggered* throughout adulthood. As a result, the individual develops behaviours and responses resulting in a recurring pattern of behaviour every time it happens; the neurological pathway that has developed over time strengthens and interferes with normal, healthy mind processes and human interaction. I believe we can change the negative response if all the steps are followed as indicated here. I have witnessed this positive outcome with my clients many times.

Creative Mind Ordering (CMO) is a technique for working with abstract pictures based on the theory of neural plasticity and art therapy that was developed by the innovative German art therapist Otto Hanus (2008).

The science behind CMO is based on research showing how neurons connect and disconnect in our brain. When two connected neurons are repeatedly triggered at the same time on several occasions (either by a person learning new knowledge or by experience), the cells and the minute gap (synapses) between them change chemically, so that when one neuron fires, it serves as a stronger trigger for the other to fire as well, and in the future, they will fire off in tandem much more readily than before (Dispenza, 2017). Consequently, we often use the saying **"Neurons that fire together, wire together"**. In the same way, it could be said, "Neurons that stop firing together, stop wiring together, and the connections eventually deteriorate and fall apart."

CMO's theoretical underpinnings makes it a technical rather than emotionally directed technique – its focus is on cause and effect relationships that need to be redirected or changed. CMO is most appropriate for clients who are very committed to therapy, with good cognitive abilities, who are verbal, intellectual to a degree and 'switched on'. However, I have used it many times successfully with other clients as well, although I needed to simplify the steps in this technique to make it work.

In this approach a client/you are asked to draw abstract images that represent:

> **Trigger** – external trigger that frequently evokes negative feelings
> **Symptom** – emotional response to the trigger
> **Inner Strength** – found in the unconscious mind through the image
> **Fusion** – merging of trigger and inner strength
> **Decision** – consolidating the merge of trigger and inner strength

1. Trigger

I am prompted to use Creative Mind Ordering (CMO) with most of my clients, when they tell me about triggers in their lives (situations or people that they can't get rid of) that leave them feeling very frustrated, angry or sad (symptom). The situation must have been **on-going**, so that the brain has established a firm connection. As the trigger appears to be the cause, I tend to discuss this first with clients. The clients then share the situation or person with me, who, in their lives, makes them feel really bad.

Think of a person in your life that you struggle with at the moment. It might be somebody you have known for a long time, and whenever you get together, you feel frustrated, angry or sad or similar emotions come up for you. You may have tried many things to change this, but you were not really successful. This would be an excellent trigger for CMO. Please write this trigger down on a piece of paper. Alternatively, you could also think of a situation that overwhelms you, and where you don't have control over your emotions. It is important that this has been going on for some time.

- **The trigger is external**, or outside of us and causes a recurring reaction or problem. The trigger activates the symptom. The trigger is something that occurs **frequently**. The trigger can be a situation or other people; something someone says or does.
- **How is it triggered?** Hopefully, the client feels the symptom clearly and is 'in touch' with the real problem. A negative feeling from an unexpected trigger can be an awful place to be, but remember that using the brain in new and diverse ways through art practice can establish new pathways and thus new ways of thinking, feeling and behaving.
- We are dealing here with cause and effect relationships in a psychological context, i.e. what must happen (trigger) for the symptom to evolve?

Drawing task: trigger picture

Draw an abstract picture of the trigger using A3 or A4 paper. Make sure there is nothing figurative in your image, as discussed in Chapter 6. Take about one hour or more doing this drawing or painting. You can use Caran d'Ache Neocolor I wax oil crayons (my preferred option for abstract work with clients), water colours or acrylic paint.

Note: Symbols should not be used, i.e. crosses, hearts, yin/yang sign, etc. Although slightly abstract, symbols are not advisable as they are not abstract enough; they are still representational, and interfere with the process. Symbols that emerge out of the unconscious are a different story.

Afterwards, mark the trigger picture, using adjectives and **write down** your descriptions. What happens for the symptom to emerge? Stay phenomenological (i.e. looking at *what is* rather than *why* it is – what **is in** the picture). Write this all down as you have done in the previous chapter. Get lots of ideas; go into detail describing the colour, the form, the movement, the relationships and the space between the colours and shapes and lines. The trick in 'art in therapy' is to describe what you see, what it looks like and how it feels rather than trying to explain what you were thinking and what it means to you, which only represents the tip of the iceberg. You can describe and mind map your trigger as you have done before with your self-picture.

Some tips for marking all the pictures

- Use adjectives, feeling words, metaphors (it reminds me of a . . .). Create associations within the pictures, discover symbols and deeper meaning (although remember the client should not deliberately 'put' symbols in the picture when drawing; the symbols should emerge out of the unconscious, but don't start looking for them either). The associations created will give you an idea of what the picture means to the client.

- We also use our framework for working with abstract drawings and paintings by looking at the forms within the picture, the use of space, the movement within it and the relationship between the parts.
- We are also interested in the feelings associated with what the client sees.
- As you describe the picture and link the client's words together, a story will form. Every picture is a story and the richer and fuller the story, the more useful it is. The therapist draws all the ideas together in a mind map, and makes sense of the pieces as a whole, in light of the picture, while being sure to check with the client if it fits for them.
- Some helpful questions: What does it remind you of? What is your overall impression? What else comes to mind when you look at the picture, the different colours, the shapes, the movement and the way the colours and shapes relate to each other? What feelings are you aware of as you look at all those aspects respectively?

Creative Mind Ordering example

Trigger picture: Tania

Rob: Please draw an abstract trigger picture of your sister, whom you are experiencing as being 'very black and white' in her thinking.

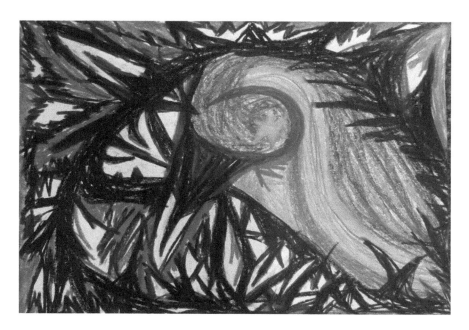

Rob: How does the image look to you?

Tania: **Colour in the centre . . . but . . . within that there is a firm, solidness . . . Something hidden/covered . . . Black and white in nature . . . inflexible . . . sharp and cutting.**

Rob: Do you have a sense of your sister being firm and when you experience your sister, are you aware that she is firm and solid in her ways?

Tania: Yes, she is very strong in her appearance. She is always right.

Rob: What do you think is covered and hidden with your sister?

Tania: I think that she gets a bit jealous of the lifestyle of others . . . she hides the fact that she has those feelings.

Rob: What is her black and white nature?

Tania: That's what drives me crazy – she doesn't see grey . . . e.g. you can't change your mind about a decision . . . inflexible.

Rob: There is a sharpness to her that is cutting?

Tania: She tries to be nice but to me she is sharp and cutting with her tongue – can cut right through your heart . . . She is tactless, always right.

Exploring the symptom

Rob: When this happens with your sister, how do you feel about it? What is the symptom for you?

Tania: I get angry and frustrated with her. I get anxious . . . Negative self-talk . . .

Rob: What negative self-talk would you do?

Tania: . . . that I should have it all together by now, but . . . see my struggle . . . I'm not good enough . . .

2.   *Symptom*

Now, I would like **you**, the reader, to think about the feelings you have when you are triggered by someone or something in your life. Most clients talk about frustration or anger towards a person or situation, but I suggest you look for feelings that are deep, such as how the person leaves you feeling, for this is the 'symptom'. Look for feelings of being strongly affected by someone, even after you have seen them, and not how you relate to him or her. For example, you might feel lost, lonely, not worthy, etc., rather than angry towards them. Please write down these feelings. This might be a bit hard to do by yourself, as the art therapist normally has a good skill in prompting and going deeper with a client. Doing this process on your own might lead you to some levels of resistance that are hard to overcome without the help of an expert. But give it a go anyway.

The symptom is an unpleasant, inhibiting or damaging emotion, or internal reaction, and the first step to changing this pattern of reacting is to ask what the symptom or problem is. This is something we don't like (it could be an idea or belief); it may not be apparent, and it can be difficult to find. **Make sure the symptom is not the trigger.** The trigger is outside of you and the symptom is a feeling, or a thought or belief, that you have. For example, the symptom could be anger, but the trigger is your boss who fired you last week.

Note: In cognitive behavioural therapy this is all clearly separated, thoughts from feelings, but when it comes to the unconscious, mess is the norm. We are going to discuss how to do CBT in an ordered way with 'messy' art therapy in the next chapter.

Drawing task: symptom picture

Please draw an abstract picture of the symptom. Take about an hour or more to do this drawing or painting, that represents your most unpleasant, disturbing or anxiety-provoking feelings, thoughts or behaviours that occur repeatedly in your life when the trigger occurs. Also, in your mind, phrase this symptom into adjectives that describes your picture in its truest sense, i.e. 'I feel . . . angry, or locked up, or sad, etc.' as opposed to 'I don't feel happy, I don't feel good, etc.'. I realise this might be easier to think of after you have done the picture, but just keep it in mind because the picture intervention should be phrased 'positively'. I'm using the word here to describe what something is, in its essence, because the unconscious cannot 'un'think, i.e. try **not** to see a white horse. *Note: This is about avoiding negations (not, don't, didn't, won't, etc.) when working with the unconscious and not about a negative experience. Our unconscious knows these too well.* So use nouns or adjectives for your picture phrase, i.e. if you are 'not happy', what are you – sad?

Beware of the trap in the symptom search: Do not go too far, do not analyse why you have done this or that (i.e. the cause of the symptom). And remember, the symptom must occur frequently.

Afterwards, mark the symptom picture, using adjectives as we have done before and write down the descriptions. What would have to happen for the symptom to emerge? Stay phenomenological (i.e. looking at **what is** rather than **why it is** – what **is in** the picture). Get lots of ideas; go into detail describing the colour, the form, the movement, the relations and the space, and describe **what you see rather than what you think**. I want you to focus on the negative feeling and what looks negative to you.

Symptom picture: Tania

Rob: Draw yourself feeling anxious, struggling and feeling you are not good enough.

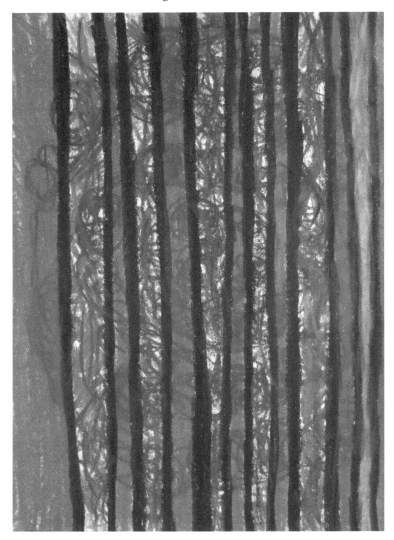

Rob: How does the image look to you?

Tania: There are lines . . . black lines down the picture.

Rob: How do they make you feel?

Tania: I feel trapped and the feeling of containment varies. Sometimes it's strong (like the wider bar), sometimes it's not as strong but there is still a barrier there . . .

Rob: What comes to mind – what is your first impression?

Tania: There's something behind it . . . it is knotted and squiggly . . . directionless.

Rob: If it doesn't have a direction, how is it?

Tania: It is all over the place.

Rob: What else comes to your mind when you think about 'trapped' and 'containment'?

Tania: It's never-ending.

Rob: How does it feel having those bars in your life?

Tania: Not free. (*Note: This is a negation, so I needed to translate it into a 'positive' formulation.*)

Rob: If you are not free, what are you?

Tania: Restricted. The colours bring up anger, frustration and smouldering.

Rob: **I imagine that when your sister is sharp, cutting, black and white, inflexible, you feel trapped, restricted and contained or confused and all over the place? Does this resonate with you?**

Tania: I feel like nothing is ever good enough and in her eyes whatever I do I will still be restricted by her ideas . . .

Rob: And how do you feel in your life?

Tania: It depends . . . there is a lot of anger, resentment and frustration . . . Even when things are not too bad, the bars move then she speaks again and 'lights the fire' and I feel anger and frustration, and smouldering.

Note: Sometimes clients, when they hear the words reflected back, realise that there is an older trigger that is stronger, like it might not be so much about the sister, but about the mother. In this case, it can be worthwhile to try the entire process again, starting with the mother as the trigger. Another example would be a boss that reminds you of your stepfather as the older and stronger trigger. Therefore, I would ask the client to draw the trigger picture again, but this time of the stepfather. Art therapy and the work with the unconscious is a dynamic process, and it is OK to go backwards and forwards at times.

Rob: **While you experience these sensations in your picture, is there an area that is not knotty and squiggly, confused and all over the place, where you are not contained and restricted by her ideas? What about the picture do you actually like, that is not connected to your negative descriptions?**

Note: I am looking now for the inner strength!
    Client points to an area of the image, the yellow on the right hand side.

Rob: Now tell me, how does this area look different to the rest?

Tania: It's clearer. It's more defined. Certain. It's more defined and its own entity. It's brighter . . .

Rob: And the shape of it, the movement in it and the position of it . . . What else stands out for you?

Tania: It's on the edge a bit . . .

Rob: How does it feel being on the edge?

Tania: OK.

Rob: How come?

Tania: Because it's still supported by the two bars . . .

Rob: Anything else?
Tania: It's unblocked . . .
Rob: And what does it mean to be unblocked?
Tania: Freer.
Rob: **What are other moments in your life where you felt bright, certain, clear, supported and free? What would that experience be?**
Tania: Riding a bike.

Note: The unconscious is advising us not to completely go into 'symptom mode' – imagine riding a bike when you are experiencing your sister behaving in a harsh and cutting way.

3.   Inner strength

We need to look for positive phenomena in your, the reader's, symptom picture, places in the picture that you actually like. I am aware that this sounds bizarre. How could there be something you like, (positive) in such a negative picture? This is one of the most amazing things about this technique. The way I understand it is like this. Our unconscious suffers from experiencing the trigger and it looks for a way out. The unconscious not only projects the problem experience into the picture when you are drawing, but also it searches for a better way to deal with the trigger and projects that as well, and this positive area is often quite small and can easily be overlooked, like a white corner, a dash of yellow on the top etc.
    There are two areas of focus in your symptom picture.

    Negative characteristics, (see above) which should be fairly obvious.
    Positive characteristics, which are more hidden and normally take up only a very small section of the whole image.

For this next part we will need the positive descriptions to do the work with the 'inner strength', so that we can create a change to the response of the trigger.
    Note: We have a lot of wisdom in us. Remember the Chapter 5 on goals, and how our unconscious would not only project 'obstacles' in the picture but also 'strength' to overcome them? Something very similar is happening here.

- Ask yourself/or your client, to point to a spot you like best in the picture (even though it is a *'negative'* picture). What is positive? What parts do you like even though it might be just a spot? Where would you like to put yourself in the picture if you were a little button or a chess figure? (I always use a pawn for this exercise, like in the Self-Box activity.) Point to an area that is not like the rest of the symptom picture and that is different to all the symptom descriptions. Describe this new found area in great detail, describing the colour and how it feels, the shape, and how it feels, the movement, and how it feels and any relationships, and how they feel, and as usual take notes. The inner resource is sitting in the picture. Good and bad can sit together quite comfortably in the unconscious, like love and hate.

- Can you find a strength in the marking of the symptom picture? A strength that you really know well about yourself?
- Look at the words that you have written down. Try not to think about the trigger or the symptom, but look at these words independently in context with your life. What situation comes to your mind when you feel like this? While you're doing the next task, please visualise the words and this situation or positive experience, e.g. riding a bike or walking a dog on the beach.

Drawing task: inner strength picture

Please draw an abstract picture of your strength (see marking and experience above). Take about one hour or more doing this drawing or painting. You can have a look below how I phrased this task for Tania before you start your drawing.

Afterwards, mark the inner strength picture, using adjectives as we have done before and write down the descriptions. Do the words ring a bell for you? Do you feel well, when you are like this? For some reason, your unconscious believes that when you are being this way, it will help you deal with the trigger. Can you see the link or is it still hard to imagine at this stage? We are not finished yet.

When we experience the symptom, our unconscious mind doesn't like it. In its wisdom, it looks for a way out – it projects something into the image that is different, something that is positive – an 'inner strength'. As the unconscious experiences, feeling trapped, restricted, confused and smouldering, the unconscious also creates an opportunity to respond in another way to the trigger, which is the inner strength.

Inner strength picture: Tania

Rob: Draw your inner strength, feeling 100% (do not think about the trigger or symptom at this stage) strong, bright, certain, clear and defined; in its own entity supported and free.

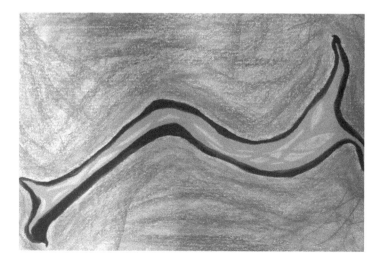

Rob: When you look at this image, how does it look to you?
Tania: It looks like it's floating . . . It's free . . .
Rob: What colour did you use?
Tania: Green, it's calm, floating . . . fluid, relaxed . . . It's still safe.
Rob: What is safe in the picture?
Tania: It has a border.
Rob: How do you feel within that border?
Tania: I feel relaxed, safe and free . . . I feel together.
Rob: And when you describe the colours how would you describe it in comparison to the other one? (Background large area).
Tania: It's defined . . . strong, but it's moving around me, it's gentle . . . I'm protected . . . . It's solid, but still allows for change inside it.

Note: Reading back to the client – In the example of the surrounding colour areas (orange/yellow) did not appear to be the main theme, as she did not mention it. The road in the image appeared to be the central theme – so I chose to finish there . . .

Rob: **In your life at the moment, you are aware of your inner strength . . . it is calming and relaxing. While you are cycling, you experience that calming, relaxing . . . and you feel free, protected and safe.**

4. Fusion

- When I ask my clients, "Can you imagine yourself responding to your trigger with your inner strength?", most of them say, "You must be mad! That is the last thing I feel when I am exposed to the trigger. How could I possibly feel like that, with that situation or that person around me?" I tell them not to worry too much about it at this stage. All they need to do next is a geometrical activity that will connect those two areas in their brain and then they might feel differently about it afterwards.
- **This is the crucial drawing used to create a new pathway.** This is where the Creative Mind Ordering will take place. By placing the trigger picture and the inner strength picture together and drawing the two pictures equally represented in a third fusion picture, the client will create a new neural pathway that connects both areas. While the client is drawing the fusion, the neurons in our brain will fire together, for both the trigger representation, and the inner strength.
- **Remember this: when neurons fire together, they wire together.**

Drawing task: fusion picture

Please draw an abstract picture of the fusion. I would like you to take the trigger picture and the strength picture and create a new image where both are represented equally – a fusion. This is more a 'geometrical' activity where you bring different elements together (shapes and colours) that may not make much sense in real life. How can the resource feeling you have come into play when you experience the trigger? Can it? Take about one hour or more doing this drawing or painting.

Afterwards, mark the fusion picture using the marking criteria, acknowledging your ability to fuse the two pictures, the trigger and the strength.

In art therapy, we move on from the marking process to assist the clients in creating a decision as to how they will respond the next time the trigger occurs. When the trigger happens again, they will be able to respond with the strength and not the symptom, e.g. when fear (trigger) occurs, then I will feel safe and protected (strength).

- Ask how the client will behave in the future when the trigger presents itself; identify a behaviour that will support him or her. After the fusion picture is drawn there is a **new** connection between the trigger and the strength. The more you use this connection and your neural pathways fire together, the more they wire together. Visualise the strength when the trigger occurs. Have the picture in front of you. Ask yourself how you will behave in the future when your trigger presents itself and write it down.
- The long-term result is that when the old neural pathways between trigger and symptom aren't used any longer, they deteriorate and disconnect (Dispenza, 2017). So when the trigger happens in the future, it won't create the symptom any longer. When I see clients much later, they often tell me with great surprise how they haven't felt the symptom any longer in context with the trigger and that they can't believe they'd ever feel this way.

Fusion picture: Tania

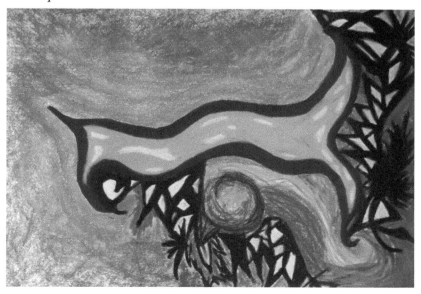

Rob: What does the image look like?

Tania: More safe. I actually feel strong when I look at the picture. I feel protected by the borders . . . she can't penetrate. Although the sharp tongue is still there, it does not make me bleed so much . . . It doesn't cut me like it did before.

Rob: If it doesn't bleed and cut you . . . what does her sharp tongue do to you in the picture?

Tania: I can deflect her . . . I can 'flick her away.' Having the calm and safety/orange protection around me I can allow bits of her to get closer to me . . . The pink feels like people can see that she is very black and white, but they can also see me 'keeping my cool' . . .

Rob: Where do you see yourself being strong in the picture?

Tania: The purple border . . .

Rob: What is it about the purple border – how does it look?

Tania: It allows me to adapt to her . . . It stands out more than my sister.

Rob: **So, I imagine that when your sister is all black and white to you, you could deflect her, or you could choose to remain strong, calm and keep your cool. When her sharp tongue hits you, you have the choice to deflect it and mentally 'flick her away', visually in your mind. At the same time when that happens you will feel safe, calm and protected by the borders. This will allow you to keep your cool. Can you see how this relates to your life?**

Tania: **Yes, I totally can.**

Homework

Meditate, consolidate and practise the connection between the trigger and the strength and when the trigger occurs visualise the strength as much as you can. These actions support developing the new neural pathways. The fusion is more believable over time and will become more established in your brain. The inner strength will have a strong neural connection to the trigger, and the trigger loses its emotional impact, because it doesn't trigger the symptom any longer.

5.   *Decision*

The decision picture will reinforce the connection in the brain. I tend to ask my clients to draw the decision picture many weeks later when they have experienced the effect of the fusion, when they have been successful in responding to the trigger with their inner strength.

- I would like you to write down what has become important in this process. Look at the marking of the fusion picture, and what decision you have made, such as "always responding with my inner strength to the trigger". Write a decision text on what has become important in this process. Look at what comes up in the fusion picture. What decision are you making? *"In the future .. .(when the trigger occurs), I will always respond . . .* (with inner strength)." It must make sense. Then come up with a decision statement, e.g. *"When I am accused of . . . (trigger) from now on I will decide to . . . (inner strength)."*

- The next step leads to a decision picture. This will be similar to the fusion picture. The significance of the inner strength will be greater and the trigger will have less significance and will hopefully not be a threat any longer. Visualise and feel that decision. It will anchor strongly in the unconscious when we draw the decision.

- Although the trigger will still be there, and we cannot deny that it could always be in our life, we are deciding to change the way we respond to it.

- *Note: The great wisdom behind CMO that we can also find in many cultures throughout the world, and even in cognitive therapy, is that the triggers in our environment are rarely the problem. The real problem is how we respond towards them and how we feel about them. Cognitive therapy would mainly target the thoughts, but our unconscious is a bit more holistic and responds in a more complex but very effective and individual way. Every client has their own way of dealing with triggers and as an outsider we have no idea what that is, so we need to be respectful and facilitate a process where the clients can find their own answers in CMO.*

- By anchoring the trigger to something positive, nurturing and grounding, we fight the disturbing inner images by thinking of a positive self and a 'powerful' experience. As the old neural pathway is not used, the symptom will correspondingly weaken. Therefore, the result is that we are aware of the trigger but no longer responding in a way that results in experiencing the old symptom or emotion. The pathway that is not used will eventually deteriorate. **The trigger won't change, but the response will be different.**

Drawing task: decision picture

Put all three pictures (trigger, symptom and fusion) and the decision text in front of you. Focus on your inner strength as an answer to the trigger in the future and for the rest of your life, and make a clear decision. In this last step, I would like you to do a fusion between your trigger and your inner strength again, but this time not just a 'geometrical' activity, but I would like you to believe in it. Believe that you can hold on to your inner strength even when the trigger occurs. This is supported by Dan Siegel's (2017, p. 179) "where attention goes, neural firing flows and neural connection grows", a clever and creative adaptation of one of the Huna Life Principles. At this point most of my clients draw their inner strength first and then add the trigger to the picture in a way that does not affect the resource negatively. There is now a kind of 'buffer' between the two, so no matter how 'nasty' or intense the trigger is, it does not affect negatively the inner strength in its core. This process will allow for stronger neural connections between the trigger and the inner strength.

Bring the main elements of the two pictures together, the trigger and the inner strength picture, to create another fusion image, the decision picture.

Afterwards, mark the decision picture using the marking criteria, take notes as usual, and acknowledge your ability to respond with your inner strength to the trigger, practising this concept whenever it comes up, and for the rest of your life.

*As the client draws this, the two areas of the brain fire together. As they "fire together, they wire together" (neuroplasticity). While the client draws this, the **new neural pathway is strengthened**.*

Decision picture: Tania

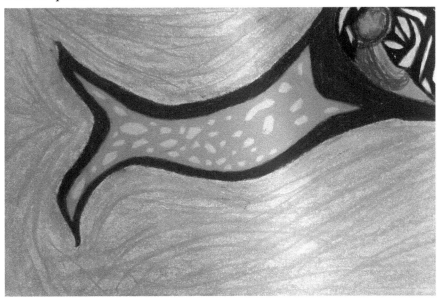

I discussed with Tania how would it be for her if every time her sister is "sharp, cutting, black and white", she remained "calm, safe and feeling strong"? We did not get to mark Tania's decision picture, but she reported how the inner strengths were becoming the dominant response towards the trigger. *Note: you can see in Figure 8.6 how it has changed in comparison to the fusion picture. This is not always as visible as it is here. Sometimes, the fusion picture is more powerful than the decision picture. Every client is different.*

Conclusion

As we take risks and experiment, we capitalise on the brain's left and right hemispheres and its capacity also for nonverbal, nonlinear experiences. Inner healing takes place because of this 'creative connection'. The creative connection process stimulates a form of self-exploration. As feelings are tapped, they become a resource for further self-understanding and creativity. We gently allow ourselves to bring forth what has been denied to awareness – that which rests in our unconscious. Simply put, we cannot integrate all aspects of the self without involving all aspects of the self.

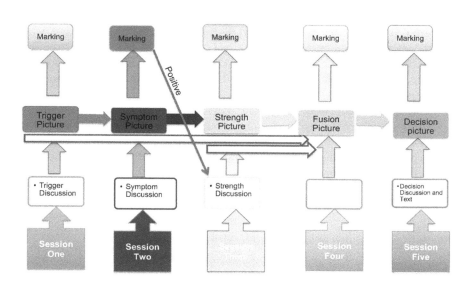

Diagram of the CMO process
* Start at the bottom with Session 1 and follow the arrows to Session 2 etc.

Creative Mind Ordering based on mechanisms of brain plasticity can change disturbing or anxiety-provoking feelings, thoughts or behaviours that occur repeatedly, to adaptive actions, and increase feelings of resilience to an external trigger, such as a person or situation.

CMO: additional points

- There are certain actions we do repetitively in relationships with parents, siblings and employers. It is a cycle that is hard to control, change or prevent, as if we are programmed to behave in a certain way. We don't know how to change our response even though we may challenge ourselves not to respond in the same way.
- **Example:** A client presents with an eating disorder (the symptom). Upon questioning, it becomes apparent that her lack of eating is related to her mother's great expectations of her (the trigger). A strong neural pathway has been forged between the client's experience of her mother's pressure upon her (the trigger) and her obsession of feeling overweight and therefore refusing to eat (the symptom). CMO aims to create a new pathway so that the trigger leads to a different place – for example, positive self-talk about being a strong woman, so that thinking of her mother no longer leads to the symptom of not eating, but feeling

strong and independent. Of course, this is only an example. Every client is different and especially their brains and brain connections.

- This technique is beneficial especially for clients who are using the same old rehearsed ways, a repetitive behaviour they can't shake or get rid of. So, the goal is to change how they interact with each other – **like a dance that changes from the tango to the cha-cha-cha**; and while doing this, new pathways are formed.
- **For this technique it is advantageous when the client has good cognitive and verbal skills, but not essential.** Start discussing with the client in detail, what the symptom could be, to identify the real problem. The client needs to be able to articulate what is happening, and be reflective of the trigger. They also need to be able to reflect on, and identify the deep-seated trigger that might cause the symptom.
- Sometimes, the first trigger the client draws is not always from the deep unconscious, e.g. the client discusses a neighbour who annoys them; however, after delving into the picture, they identify an older trigger, the father that hurt them deeply. The neighbour might only remind them of the father. If this happens, I get the client to draw the picture again.
- If your clients do not have these skills, you might still be able to use CMO, but you need to adjust it to the capacity of your client.

Warning: when not to use Creative Mind Ordering

This technique is used mainly for clients who can't change their triggers. Often, triggers get too much negative attention, and are not that bad after all. Sometimes, all a client needs is more resilience. The spiritual or philosophical idea is that often our responses to a situation are the problem, rather than external factors or triggers.

However, if a trigger is really bad or harmful, such as an abusive relationship, our first goal is to stop the external problem from continuing, and not in helping the client to learn to live with it. The most important principle in the Code of Conduct, which I was taught during my psychology degree, is "First, do no harm". Therefore, you need to consider if the situation can be changed or if the thinking and response to it is the main problem. Otherwise, we condone the abuse, and the problem with this technique is that it really works, so our clients would be enabled to 'put up' with abuse.

Literature

Chia-Shu, L., Yong, L., Wei-Yuan, H., Chia-Feng, L., Shin, T., Tzong-Ching, J., Yong, H., Yu-Te, W., Tianzi, J. & Jen-Chuen, H. (2013, June). Sculpting the intrinsic modular organization of spontaneous brain activity by art. Retrieved 23 May 2018 from https://doi.org/10.1371/journal.pone.0066761

Dispenza, J. (2017). *Becoming supernatural: How common people are doing the uncommon.* California: Hay House.

Hanus, O. (2008). *Creative paths to solutions* (trans.). Nordestedt: Books on Demand.

Lorenz, M. (2006, July). Stress and psychoneuroimmunology revisited: Using mind-body interventions to reduce stress. Retrieved 23 May 2018 from www.mm3admin.co.za/documents/docmanager/6e64f7e1-715e-4fd6-8315-424683839664/00025132.pdf

Malchiodi, C. (2012). Art therapy and the brain. In C. Malchiodi (Ed.), *Handbook of art therapy* (2nd Ed.), (pp. 17–26). New York: The Guildford Press.

Malchiodi, C. (2013, August). Art therapy and mild traumatic brain injury. My personal experience with a mild TBI and why art helps. Retrieved 23 May 2018 from www.psychologytoday.com/us/blog/arts-and-health/201308/art-therapy-and-mild-traumatic-brain-injury

Siegel, D.J. (2017). *Mind: A journey to the heart of being human*. New York, London: Norton.

CHAPTER 9

Advancing art therapy and cognitive behaviour therapy (CBT)

Psychology may be a science, but psychotherapy is an art.

In this chapter I would like to present an example showcasing how many psychologists work and how to effectively bring in art therapy, showing art therapy at its finest and not just as a nice decoration, or a form of entertainment while the therapist is thinking about what to do next. Art therapy is the external representation of our thoughts, and bringing together the functions of thinking with the representation of art allows people to think more powerfully (Kirsh, 2010), to gain a deeper understanding of themselves.

There are over 500 psychotherapy treatments that are practised in the world (Pearsall, 2011). Cognitive behavioural therapy or CBT is still the most widely used.

Many clients, however, cannot attend appointments due to financial or physical challenges and some struggle cognitively or verbally. Morris (2014) speaks about an integration of CBT with art therapy that could benefit clients who otherwise do not respond well with CBT alone. In conventional CBT, clients are required to visualise and verbalise ideas. As art therapy has methods that works with the unconscious, the integration of art therapy with CBT creates the possibility of a brief intervention model with long lasting outcomes, a win-win situation for both.

Huss (2013) notes the fundamental difference between art making and CBT is the 'location' of the image – in other words, whether the idea or problem is imagined in the mind (CBT) or is viewed as a concrete, physical image (art therapy), they both function to serve the same purpose.

Note: If you are not a psychologist or just not familiar with CBT, it might be very useful to read up on this area of psychology before studying this chapter. There is so much on the Internet about CBT and in your local book store/ library. This extremely valuable approach in psychotherapy should be known to any clinician, including art therapists.

When learning about CBT, as an art therapist, I recommend focusing on the topics around positive and negative reinforcement, role modelling, fear hierarchy, gradual exposure and desensitization, relaxation training, the ABC of rational–emotive therapy (RET) and how to achieve a change of core beliefs, schemas, assumptions, attributions and cognitions in general, and as a personal treat, mindfulness-based cognitive therapy.

The very basic premise of CBT is that emotions are a result of thought, which then affects behaviour. Through CBT a client can learn what part of their thinking needs to change in order to affect their feelings and behaviour. **However, on its own, CBT is not without pitfalls. Clients need to first find out what they really think and feel, on a deeper level, something that art therapy does extremely well. The externalised representations, unconscious projections and underlying cognitions and feelings can be made conscious through art therapy.**

According to Hofmann and Asmundson (2008), there are six steps to carrying out CBT, and these steps have been used to form six or seven sessions of CBT. The *Management of Mental Disorders Manual* (Andrews et al., 2013) lists four key factors of CBT. The first is to explain the rationale behind cognitive behaviour therapy – psychoeducation. Then identify negative or irrational thoughts. Test these thoughts – evidence for and against, how likely are they? And, finally, challenge these cognitions and generate more rational and realistic thoughts.

In my experience, many CBT therapists are struggling today, as they feel something is missing to make a long-lasting impact. I know several CBT therapists in the United States, who do long term CBT (yes, that exists) and who feel the need to tap into unconscious or underlying cognitions. There is a strong belief among art therapists that art therapy can enhance traditional CBT and that CBT-based art therapy may be as effective as psychodynamic-based approaches (Rosal, 2001). It is most probable that no single definitive approach will ever be adequate to cover the complexity of individual client needs, so adding CBT to art therapy, and vice versa, might be the secret ingredient that makes a difference.

Part of the problem with only using CBT is that medical metaphors pervade psychological literature, which often frames the way therapists might use language with their clients to conceptualise their problem or illness. Metaphors, in general, do help us to see thoughts in a different light, however we are still limited to a talking-therapy, and research suggests that visual cues help us to retrieve and remember information. Psychotherapy would be better enhanced with disciplines of creative expression rather than being 'stuck' in a medical paradigm. Nevertheless, CBT appears to be the most evidence-based treatment strategy in psychotherapy across various client groups and psychiatric disorders, as indicated in several meta-analyses (Hofmann et al., 2012), so art therapists can remain critical but need to be open to it as well. Likewise, those who are CBT-based need to see the advantage of visual work and the work with the unconscious as the client may develop more positive ideas on how to behave in a certain situation by experimenting first on paper on a deeper level rather than being overwhelmed with the real situation.

There are quite a few CBT therapists that include other approaches that have become popular over the last few years. Comer (2015) labeled them New Wave within the CBT framework, and I normally like to call them "CBT and Mindfulness Approaches" stemming from an spiritual tradition. One of my favourites is mindfulness-based cognitive therapies (MBCT), which has a contemplative approach to therapy and is often used for depression, stress and anxiety issues or disorders. If you work with borderline personality disorders or any other mental health issues, e.g. clients who engage in suicidal behaviour, you have probably come across dialectical behavioural therapy (DBT), which combines CBT with mindfulness skills. Another popular variant, is motivational interviewing (MI), that is particularly used in drug and alcohol counselling, but can also be helpful in other contexts. Acceptance and commitment therapy (ACT) has also become quite popular over the last years and can be used for all sorts of issues. I believe we not only enhance the methods, but we have better client outcomes if we use art therapy in conjunction with CBT, and any of the therapies mentioned here.

If you'd like more information about these approaches you can search the net, or enrol on a short-term course or workshop. It will definitely be worth your while.

CBT can be a nice addition to the art therapy tool box and very useful on the therapeutic journey, so now, let's have a look at how we can do CBT as an art therapist, or how we can do art therapy as a cognitive behaviour therapist.

Advancing art therapy and CBT

A process in eight sequences with six images

I would like to acknowledge the creative ideas of the German art therapist Otto Hanus (2008) who developed this technique. I have used many of his ideas in the specific approach that I am showcasing here, but I have also changed some aspects to suit practising psychologists and art therapists alike.

Note for psychologists: If you don't have much time to go through all the sequences with your client, (the sad reality of many clinicians), you could just use this first sequence to find the underlying thought and continue with traditional CBT.

Note for art therapists: If you also would like to short-cut this technique, I recommend doing only picture 1, picture 2 and picture 6. This is what I tend to do with most of my clients. It is a great luxury to take time, it makes a lot of sense to take things slowly, but our clients might have a different agenda, after all.

Note for readers: I think it is a good idea if you do all the exercises and pictures, so you can decide what parts work for you and which ones you would like to omit, if any. I keep changing my approach and what I teach all the time. Certainly, copy what you read in this book, but also make it yours, change it organically, utilise what you already have and transform into the art therapist you want to become.

Sequence 1: unwanted cognition

1   **Communication**: Which cognitions, thoughts, attitudes, beliefs or attributes do you want to change? Often clients find their unwanted thought by first looking at situations they don't like, for example, a domineering boss or a neighbour who has started ignoring them. These situations might make them feel sad or angry, but as you might have picked up in the readings about Albert Ellis's ABC (1957), it is not the situation that makes you angry or sad, but what you think about it. Now, ask yourself, what thinking do you have that makes you angry, frustrated, sad or anxious around others or specific situations. This is the unwanted cognition we want to change.

1   *We can't do any of the communications in the following sequences with each other while you read the book, so you need to have an internal dialogue with yourself instead, and come up with something by yourself! Please write down what comes to mind in each sequence. Perhaps, you can talk to a friend, or a partner, about this before you decide what unwanted cognition you want to change.*

2   **Abstract image instruction**: The client is asked to draw an experience of their unwanted cognition as an abstract image.

3   **Abstract image**: Picture 1 – unwanted cognition (*please draw this image now; take about 30–60 minutes approximately*).

4   **Marking**: If the client expresses their unwanted cognition in this image, how do they experience it? This would be the question to ask your clients. During this process *write down the descriptions of your image, and the associations that you have with it. I call this the 'marking' of an image and please do this for all the following sequences.* We are trying to uncover the underlying deeper cognitions if there are any. Something CBT can't do without working with the unconscious, i.e. art therapy.

Example: unwanted (negative) cognition conversation with Ana

Ana: I have trouble meeting new people and often avoid them. When I meet new people, I always feel anxious and scared about what they are going to say or do to me.

Rob: Can you come up with some words to describe what you are thinking when you feel anxious and scared around new people?

Ana: I'm thinking . . . that I'm not as good as them, small, downsized, and insignificant . . . when I meet new people.

I asked Ana to draw the essence of her unwanted cognition, *being small, downsized and insignificant.*

Ana's drawing

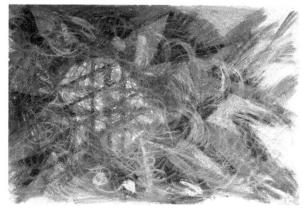

Rob: What's your first impression, when you're looking at your picture?

Ana: It's messy, which I didn't expect.

Rob: Yes, what else?

Ana: Ummm, it's cloudy or clouded over, as if it's disappearing, the behind part is disappearing, and it's a feeling of . . . well it's sort of layered, and that was intentional because underneath, there were all these points of attack, all these triangles underneath, that were attacking this kind of central part, this yellow part . . .

Rob: So these triangles, underneath, describe how they can attack you?

Ana: Well these very sharp triangles came in and attacked, the centre, but then I covered them over. So it looks messy . . .

Rob: So, basically, the experience for you, it's a mess, you feel messy inside . . .

Ana: Yes.

Rob: And you also feel like you're disappearing . . .

Ana: Yes.

Rob: . . . because your centre is being attacked . . .

Ana: Yes.

Rob: From somewhere . . . a place that comes from underneath. It's not obvious, the attack is coming from underneath but it's getting to your centre, and makes you feel like you disappear.

Ana: Yes.

Rob: So the experience feels like something from underneath is attacking you in a sharp way that makes you disappear. What is happening at the moment or what else happened in your life that resembles that? Being attacked from underneath, in a sharp way that makes it very messy for you, and you start disappearing? What experience comes to mind?

Ana: Ever since I migrated to this country, I didn't feel a sense of belonging. It was a big contrast going to school here in Australia, that was very, very hard . . . I didn't know the language very well, I couldn't speak English, and I remember one time, asking a student next to me, 'What did the teacher say?' And I got into trouble and the teacher called me over, I was about six years old and she caned me in front of the class, with a very sharp object, a large wooden toy block. It really hurt.

Rob: What was going on for you? What were you thinking?

Ana: So I felt very . . . like I couldn't work out what I did wrong.

Rob: Ah, that's why, so that's basically what it is, that experience, that you haven't done anything wrong but she (the teacher) misunderstood the situation and could not communicate what was wrong and in those days you got caned for just looking in the wrong direction.

Ana: That's right.

Rob: So for you it was very confusing, and you probably felt like you didn't do anything wrong, but you got caned.

Ana: So, there must be something wrong about me. Ah, that's how I feel small, insignificant and stupid when I meet new people.

Rob: So you deserve this, in a way.

Ana: Yeah.

Rob: So in your life, wherever you go, in new situations especially, you expect being insignificant and stupid and getting attacked.

Ana: Makes sense!

Rob: And because of that expectation of being attacked in any new situation because you are insignificant and stupid, you might avoid new situations and people in general.

Ana: That's right. I don't like meeting new people at all, at all.

Rob: So consequence is (writes this down) 'Don't . . . like . . . meeting new people'.

Ana: And I also hate losing friends; if I've lost a friend, I feel worse.

Rob: Like when you lost your friends in Poland, that gave you a different experience of yourself when you were not downsized, small, insignificant and stupid. So your cognition is 'my old contacts are good, I don't want to lose them, my new contacts are going to attack me because I'm 'insignificant, small, downsized and stupid'. That's your thinking, and it really worries and scares you when you meet new people.

Ana: I agree!

Rob: And that thinking does not help you.

Ana: No.

Rob: Now we understand where your thinking comes from, and we can change that thinking if you wish.

Note: Because a cognitive therapist isn't able to know that a client has certain thoughts, like "There is something wrong with me", underlying their issue of not being able to make new friends which is producing their negative feelings, they might say, "OK so, let's talk about how we make friends", and never discover that first critical experience. This is where the work with the unconscious and art therapy transcends.

Sequence 2: doubt

We want to create doubt about the belief we have around a negative experience. Though a negative experience may have happened many times to reinforce that belief, for the purpose of changing this cognition we need to find the exceptions and create doubt. You may want to look at the conversation I had with Ana, first (see below), before trying to create your own doubts.

1   **Communication**: Looking at the first picture, ask the client what is he or she doubtful of, in relation to the issue? Which doubts stand out? During this communication, write down the client's doubts, or for yourself, write down your doubts. As this is a very involved exercise in cognitive therapy and you might find it difficult to do on your own, you might need a friend or a psychotherapist to help you to find some doubts.

The art therapist can ask – What is the evidence of this unwanted cognition? Is the evidence actually true? Eventually, the client starts to understand that there is very little evidence, that there are many exceptions, and the client starts to doubt their negative cognition. However, clients at the start of therapy are often convinced that there is plenty of evidence that supports their negative cognition and that it is true. This is where a lengthy discussion may be required, and the cognitive therapist needs to be assertive in order to help the client produce doubt.

Note: There are short workshops in cognitive or advanced cognitive therapy, for all art therapists, and I highly recommend doing one of them. This is about increasing our skills and does not mean that you necessarily follow the CBT paradigm. Personally speaking, it never sits well with me to disagree with clients and persuade them of anything. Alternatively, when we are aiming for doubt in our clients, we can also allow the client to take the leadership, becoming his or her own main critic.

2   **Abstract image instruction**: The client should create an abstract image of the experience of doubt, but the image needs to be 'stronger' than the first picture of the unwanted cognition; it needs to be convincing, so the doubt can 'take over', *i.e. colours with more depth, more substance overall; this is where it helps when you are an artist or you understand art.*

3   **Abstract image**: Draw – Picture 2 – Doubt: I have found three options that I use with my clients:

   a   Doubt about my negative cognition, e.g. There is something wrong with me (this would be the classic approach) – draw a picture of, 'doubting that there is something wrong with you'.

   b   Doubt about what comes up, because of my negative cognition, e.g. Because I feel there is something wrong with me, I should not make new friends – draw a picture of 'doubting that you should not make new friends'.

   c   Greatest personal doubt in life – draw a picture of your greatest doubt. Here we want the clients to get in touch with doubting, that nothing is for sure, including their negative cognition.

4   **Marking**: If the client experiences their doubt in this image, how do they experience it? *Describe in detail and write down your descriptions and associations.*

   If the image and the marking is not convincing, you would need to talk more to your client to create stronger doubt *(cognitive therapy)*, and then ask the client to draw it again, making it stronger, more tangible than picture 1. Therapy takes time and we are doing this to make a difference and not just ticking off a shopping list. Even if it takes many sessions, it will be worth your while at the end of the day.

Example: conversation with Ana about creating doubt

Rob: Is this really true? Is there evidence that this is really happening to you every time? Are new people always attacking you from underneath, so you start disappearing? Or are there any exceptions when new people have not attacked you? Can you find examples when new people have treated you as if there is something wrong with you and you were small, insignificant and stupid?

Ana: Well, of course, there were some people in my life that I met that didn't attack me or treat me badly.

Rob: Tell me . . . one who stands out for you straight away and who did not attack you from underneath and who was new for you.

Ana: A week ago my boss sent me a new assistant, and I told her I don't want a new assistant. I said I'll be really cranky if you send anyone.

Rob: Of course you said that, because you were thinking she is going to attack you.

Ana: She was really great.

Rob: How come, what was great about her?

Ana: I told the new person, how I didn't want an assistant and that I was cranky with my boss for sending her, and she said she liked the way I was so honest and down to earth, and she even told me she liked me.

Rob: Write that down somewhere. The message I want to bring to you, is that even though you did not want a new assistant, because of your bad unwanted cognition (I'm going to get hurt by new people because they're going to see me as downsized, small, insignificant and stupid, and it's going to be from underneath, somehow, it's going to be sharp, getting into my centre). But the experience was actually very different. She thought you are an honest person, you are down to earth, and she even said she liked you. Come on!

Ana: (*laughs*). OK.

Rob: So Ana, this cognition is actually not true. Now you are creating doubt. When you were a little girl and you came to that classroom and you got caned for no reason. That's underlying your cognition. Today, you're having some different experiences. So we're bringing doubt into this belief of 'not being good enough'. New people can actually be great. Can you see that difference?

Ana: Oh, absolutely.

Rob: So the next picture is about you having this doubt. The cognition is 'I'm not good enough and new people are going to hurt me', and you're going to doubt that. But the picture needs to be stronger than the first picture. So in this new picture you might focus more on the . . .?

Ana: Yellow. That is not disappearing by clouds.

Rob: The yellow and you being down to earth and you being honest, you being likeable. That is the new picture task for you.

Ana: Yes.

Note: We should ask for more and more examples of doubt to make the doubt even stronger, and write down the descriptions, but for the purpose of condensing the interview above it has been kept brief.

Ana's doubt picture

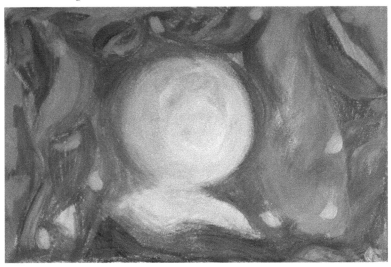

Rob: Tell me about your doubt picture.

Ana: Well I'm really happy with the yellow centre, which is bright and strong and the brown and green show my down-to-earth nature, and it feels very harmonious. It's a nice, interesting pattern and all the colours and shapes work well with each other. They look like they are interacting, and there's gentleness about it.

Rob: Does it feel like you are not good enough?

Ana: No, it doesn't. It feels like I'm in harmony with others, I'm not being attacked, the colours are floating around my yellow centre in a playful way and it feels like they like me.

Sequence 3: fusion of unwanted cognition with doubt

1   **Abstract image instruction**: The client should combine/fuse picture 1 (unwanted cognition) with picture 2 (doubt), a fusion, as we have done in Creative Mind Ordering. *Note: As you get better at this, you will start mixing techniques in a very creative, but selective way.* Your task is to get the elements of both pictures in a third picture and you have to negotiate the space on the page, as you end up with only half the space for each image. It is a rather geometrical task at the beginning, but, psychologically speaking, while you are fusing it together in the picture, thanks to our neuroplasticity, the areas in your brain communicate with each other and 'wire together'. So, we are physically bringing doubt into our negative cognition. *How amazing is that?*

2 **Fusion image**: Picture 3 – fusion of picture 1 (unwanted cognition) with picture 2 (doubts). *(Please draw this image now; take about 30–60 minutes approximately)*.

3 **Marking**: How do the doubts affect the unwanted cognition, if it (the cognition) looks like this image? Describe it in detail. Please take notes as before.

Ana's fusion picture

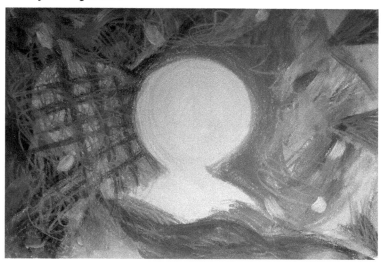

Rob: Tell me about your fusion picture. How do the doubts affect the unwanted cognition?

Ana: It's like the messy bits are behind me. They seem to be in the past because, as the yellow centre, I feel strong and vibrant, and in harmony with the other colours, so the unwanted cognition, the messy, covered over yellow, which is to the left of the picture, is still there but it doesn't have the same impact. The sharp things that were attacking my yellow centre are also not attacking anymore. They just look like they are passive.

Rob: So the doubt is strong.

Ana: Yes, the unwanted cognition, that I'm not good enough, and that new people will hurt me, doesn't have the same impact because of the doubt. In fact, it seems there is a lot of strength in the centre and the outside messy bits work harmoniously.

Sequence 4: wanted cognition

1 **Communication**: Which different (new) cognitions/attitudes, beliefs or attributes should replace the unwanted one *(no negation allowed: what do you*

want and not what you don't want)? We are using cognitive therapy here in the classical sense. We need to support our client to discover a new cognition, but remember that it should come from the client and not us. The pictures so far should help the client to find a new cognition more easily. *You might want to discuss this again with a friend who can help you to come up with an alternative and more helpful cognition.*

2   **Abstract image instruction**: The client is asked to draw an abstract image of the alternative cognition and how it looks in their life.

3   **Abstract image**: Picture 4 – wanted cognition. (*Please draw this image now; take about 30–60 minutes approximately.*)

4   **Marking**: If clients experience their wanted cognition in this image, how do they experience it? *Describe in detail and write down ideas and associations.*

Ana's wanted cognition drawing

After some discussion, Ana wanted to replace her old thinking and see herself as *assertive, significant, intelligent, and resilient.*

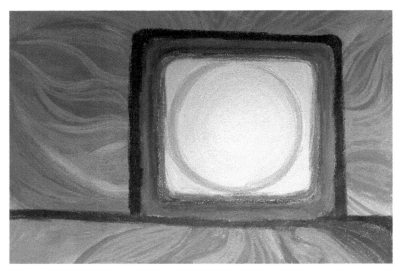

Ana: I would like to feel assertive around people. When I look at my picture, I feel as though I am strong, and very significant with that blue border and the shining yellow centre. The blue is a colour I associate with intelligence and strength. The flowing colours of pink and yellow are around me but also flowing out of me, as though I am affecting the environment. I'm in contrast to the background, but that gives me a feeling of being able to be myself in any circumstance, or to be different, so that I can speak out, and say what I want to say. The resilience is in the blue border, which is protecting my inner self, the yellow, and the way it sits on the horizon, shows me that I'm grounded, as well. (*Note: You will find that with some clients you don't need to ask many questions after some sessions, as they start to relate descriptions and ideas to their lives straight away while they are describing their picture. It's an 'all in one process'.*)

Sequence 5: positive consequences

This is a bit like the miracle question in brief solution-focused therapy (google this if you are not familiar with it)

1   **Communication**: Which positive effects or consequences could occur with this change of cognition? Think how different your life would be with this new way of thinking. Take time to look at different situations and how it could be changed if you let go of the unwanted cognition and replaced it with the new cognition. *Take notes as usual.*
2   **Abstract image instruction**: The client draws an abstract image of the new positive consequences happening in their lives.
3   **Abstract image**: Picture 5 – positive consequences. *(Please draw this image now; take about 30–60 minutes approximately.)*
4   **Marking**: If the client experiences the positive consequences in this image, how do they experience it? *Describe in detail (please take notes, as before).*

Ana's positive consequences

Ana: If I could be more assertive with people, significant and resilient, then the outcome would definitely be one of calm, and a feeling of accomplishment. It would also help me to be focused and have a more extraordinary life.

Ana's positive consequences picture

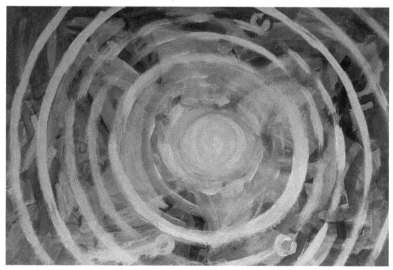

Ana: In the picture the white dominates the exciting background. The top layer of white is calming and focused in the centre. At first, I thought that I can't be calm and extraordinary at the same time. It's one or the other. But both exist in the picture together. I find the picture calming and exciting, and realise that the extraordinary in my life would be very calming. That if I allowed myself to be more assertive and resilient, I will achieve more, be more accomplished, more focused and calm, and feel better about meeting new people.

Sequence 6: fusion of wanted cognition and positive consequences

1 **Abstract image instruction**: The client combines/fuses picture 4 (wanted cognition) with picture 6 (positive consequences).
2 **Fusion image**: Picture 6 – fusion of the wanted cognition (picture 4) with positive consequences (picture 5). *(Please draw this image now; take about 30–60 minutes approximately.)*
3 **Marking**: How could this resource affect your future if it looks like this image? *Describe in detail (please take notes).*

Ana's fusion picture of sequence 4 and 5

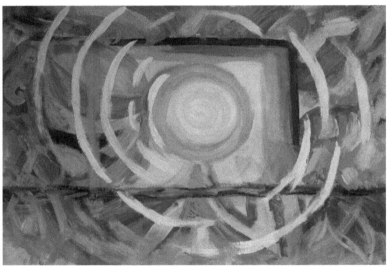

Ana: My future looks bright and happy. It radiates, communicates, connects, the background to the foreground, and it shows calm and strength, focus and flow.

Sequence 7: review

Review all sequences with a friend (or with your client) by using the images.

   Note: As I mentioned at the start, I often just do pictures 1,2 and 6 with my clients to save time. Of course, picture 6 always needs a bit more work, as we first have to explore verbally the wanted cognition and the positive consequences before the client can draw the fusion.

Picture 1 Unwanted (underlying) cognition
Picture 2 Doubt (needs to be strong)
Picture 3 Fusion of unwanted cognition with doubt
Picture 4 Wanted cognition
Picture 5 Positive consequences
Picture 6 Fusion of wanted cognition with positive consequences

Sequence 8

If the integration is achieved, traditional CBT can be used to consolidate the changes. If the integration is only partially achieved, traditional CBT can be used to do some further work with the **new conscious cognitions**. If you have skipped pictures 3–5, you could also go back. Art therapy is rarely a linear process, even though this very technical approach suggests it.

Art therapy and cognitive behaviour therapy throughout this book

I hope it has become clear in this chapter that art therapy can add value and enhance the traditional CBT approach. In the same vein, CBT can often advance art therapy. If you look back through most of the chapters in this book, you might find that I have come up with CBT interventions following the art therapy. This approach of combining art therapy and CBT works really well with clients. It would be a great asset to clinicians if this method became evidence-based practice one day.

Art therapy and CBT in these chapters

Chapter 2: We ask the client to investigate their early childhood resources and when they have found them to practise them as much as needed (CBT).
Chapter 4: We ask the client to practise their new or alternative Life Script to an extreme degree (CBT).
Chapter 6: We ask the client to focus on their strength rather their obstacles and think and behave accordingly (CBT).
Chapter 8: We ask the client to practice their inner strength in the face of their trigger (CBT).
Chapter 9: We combined art therapy and CBT throughout the entire chapter to showcase a harmonious intertwining of methods. This harmony of methods can go, of course, beyond CBT and involve other methods, like narrative therapy or working in a different context, like working with groups.

Literature

Andrews, G., Dean, K., Genderson, M., Hunt, C., Mitchell, P., Sachdev, P.S., & Trollor, J.N. (2014). *Management of mental disorders* (5th ed). Sydney: Createspace Independent Publishing Platform.

Comer, R.J. (2015). *Abnormal psychology* (9th ed.). New York: Worth.

Ellis, A. (1957). Rational psychotherapy and individual psychology. *Journal of Individual Psychology 13*, 38–44.

Hanus, O. (2008). *Creative paths to solutions* (trans.). Nordestedt: Books on Demand.

Hofmann, S.G., Asnaani, A., Vonk, I.J.J., Sawyer, A.T., & Fang, A. (2012). The efficacy of cognitive behavioral therapy: A review of meta-analyses. *Cognitive Therapy and Research 36*, 427–440.

Huss, E. (2013). *What we see and what we say: Using images in research, therapy, empowerment, and social change.* New York: Routledge.

Kirsch, D. (2010, February). Thinking with external representations. Retrieved January 15, 2019 from https://philpapers.org/archive/KIRTWE.pdf

Morris, J. (2014). Should art be integrated into cognitive-behavioral therapy for anxiety disorders. *The Arts in Psychotherapy 41*, 343–352.

Pearsall, P. (2011). *500 therapies: Discovering a science for everyday living.* New York: Norton.

Rosal, M. (2001). Cognitive-behavioural art therapy. In J. A. Rubin (Ed.), *Approaches to art therapy: Theory and technique* (2nd ed., pp. 210-226). New York: Brunner- Routledge.

CHAPTER **10**

Group art therapy

One of the most common beliefs that separates us socially and culturally is the belief that we are so different from each other that we can't possibly share our deepest feelings or be understood. Though uniqueness is intrinsic in every individual, in group art therapy, a focus takes place that allows a connectedness, where a person can feel less separated, as similar experiences and viewpoints are shared, of 'that has happened to me' or 'I feel this too'. Though this might not always happen for everyone, or at all times, group art therapy can at some point unlock for an individual the understanding that we are not alone, that our deepest fears can be shared, and that others do empathise.

If you're used to working with groups and confident of group dynamic processes, or you love enabling people to get the best out of themselves; welcoming diversity and the energy you can find in groups, you will find this chapter of great benefit. If you are a psychologist or a psychotherapist who usually works one on one, this chapter might be a perfect introduction to how you can use a group format with your clients, perhaps once a week or fortnight. If you are an artist who has been teaching art for years but wants to move into the world of psychotherapy and counselling, this might be your chapter as well.

There have been many discussions about art therapy group processes and procedures. Skaife and Huet (1998), Liebmann (2004), McNeilly (2005), Case and Dalley (2014) and Waller (2014), reflected on the effectiveness of group art therapy implemented in specific ways. Some focused more on short-term and others more on long-term group therapy sessions. Six approaches stood out for me:

1   Open groups
2   Closed groups
3   Directive groups
4   Non-directive groups
5   Thematic groups
6   Analytic groups

Another helpful distinction that could be added here is if the group is more about art as therapy or also facilitates art in therapy/ art psychotherapy (Malchiodi, 2007, 2012; Ulman, 2016).

As an art therapist, I would like to be as open and non-directive as I can be. As a psychologist, I have the need to be more clinically structured, so I can get to the bottom of the issues of my group members in a timely fashion. I know that sounds horrible for some of my readers, but the timely fashion can also mean years of group therapy with a clear focus, rather than a 'wishy-washy' approach where none of us really know what we are doing. If my main goal is art as therapy, a non-directive approach seems appropriate. If I work with a clinical population, e.g. people with diagnosed depression, I tend to become more directive in my approach, and art in therapy always follows the drawing process.

In the last 25 years of doing art in therapy with groups, there has been only one clinical and well-structured approach that stood out for me, and I use it now in every single group. I have not come across this approach in any art therapy book so far, and will focus on it here for the entire chapter.

I call this technique the Group Mural, and it was designed by the well-respected German art therapist Flora von Spreti (Spreti, Martius & Foerstl, 2012). She developed this approach while working as an art therapist in a research psychiatric hospital for over 30 years. I have found the Group Mural works really well with most groups that art therapists encounter. This approach can be used in an open or closed group format, it is very directive, has clear themes and encourages unconscious content to emerge.

The Group Mural

This is a group activity whereby each person does a drawing on their own and then shares their picture with the others in an unconventional way. The drawings are placed together on a wall or board in the form of a mural.

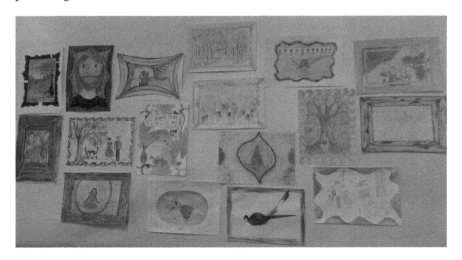

I would like you/the artist, to do this picture by yourself and then later on imagine that you are part of this art therapy group.

Time: Normally 1–2 hours for the art activity plus 1 hour for the group discussion.

Materials: Paper (A4 and A3), water colours, acrylic paint, oil crayons and colour pencils.

Instructions

1   **Picture frame**
    Each person is to draw or paint a picture frame of their choice on a piece of paper. The frame can be designed to look like it is made of metal, or timber, or it can be ornamental, modern, recycled, art nouveau, etc. You have any choice of colour, texture, material, size etc.
2   **Inside the frame: what is important to you?**
    Each person is to draw what is important to them inside the frame.

Group rules and confidentiality

After the group has finished all the drawings, and before we start with the art in therapy, I always discuss group rules, especially if the group meets for the first time or there are some new members. I normally let the group find their own rules if we have enough time. Here are a few suggestions: only one person talks at a time, be respectful towards others, be honest, be yourself, show that you care and keep it confidential.

Combining the pictures to create the Group Mural

When everyone has finished their pictures, I ask two of the group members to collect them all and create a picture composition to form a *mural* on the wall or white board. I might also ask some of the members to form a half circle with the chairs facing the mural. This is a special moment where the group members come together examining each other's artwork. Case and Dalley (2014) described it as being a moment where the unconscious of each member can affect the others, while exploring the images and how they have dealt with the theme of the day. For some it can even be a physical moment and many emotions can be elicited like, pleasure, fright, connection, etc. (Case & Dalley, 2014).

1.   Choose someone else's picture

To start the ball rolling, I ask someone in the group, whom I call the 'viewer' to choose a picture from the mural and share their viewpoint. It needs to be someone else's picture, not their own. A picture that they find interesting, enjoy, like something about, or talks to them in some way. The 'viewer' then tells the group what made them choose this image, why they like it, etc. The person who has drawn the picture we will call the 'artist'. There is a different process involved in doing a picture to looking at a picture (Wilson & Betensky, 2016).

Doing this process on your own

You/the artist, can choose a friend or family member, to be the 'viewer' and ask them to tell you what they see in your picture, what is interesting for them, possibly without taking into account that you have made it; I know that's tricky. Please write down their descriptions, what they have said.

Projections

These are 'projections' of the viewer, their comments and not necessarily what the artist/you have intended. *Note: If you are not sure what projections are, they are displaced unconscious thoughts or feelings of an individual who attributes this onto another person or thing, through a verbal comment, either negative or positive. Normally, projections are seen as something displaced and negative, but here they are 'harvested'.*

We want to capitalise on the fact that the projections of the viewers can lead to deeper insights in them and also affect the artists positively. I normally discourage clinicians from making comments to their clients about their images, as their projections or generalisations may distract the client from what is going on inside of them. In the mural technique however, I allow for the projections or comments between the group members to occur, to maximise the group effect.

Group interaction is a complex process and dependent on a range of variables including the environment, the age of the people, their cultural and socio-economic backgrounds, mental health issues, etc., but for the most part people thrive when they are part of social settings as it gives them a sense of belonging. I have observed that the underlying nature of many groups is to make comments. If you go to a barbecue for example, a common place in Australia to socialise, you will find that people comment on all sorts of things during a discussion. Someone might share with the group that her partner lost his job. Now, you can expect all kinds of responses to this like, "that job wasn't good anyway . . .", and, ". . . with his horrible boss, believe me he is better off now!" to, "I feel so sorry for you, and I still remember how devastating that was for my husband when he was made redundant". People like to make comments, and give their opinion, while showing their concern for others and unknowingly projecting their own issues.

With the mural technique, we allow projections through our comments, the good and the bad ones, just like we do in real life, but in an orderly fashion. We are actually using these projections purposefully, and in a safe manner. It can only be safe if we aim to ensure that the artists and their stories are not affected negatively, but are enhanced, instead. I'll explain how this is done.

2. Ask the viewer how the descriptions relate to his or her life

Note: This is an important step, because it allows the viewer to have some personal insights. The viewers of other pictures can discover something that they might struggle finding in their own artwork. At the same time, it has become quite clear to the group and the artist of the picture, that what the viewers are seeing in the artist's picture, is actually about themselves. This is the nature of projection.

Back to the reader of this book and the viewer you have chosen

So, is . . . and . . . (put all the descriptions from your notes in a sentence) a good description of what is happening in your life right now?

This is where the viewer might get quite surprised and have an insight into what is happening for them. Basically, we are not interested in the artist's perspective at this stage at all. We are working with the viewer of the picture and their projections. They basically see what is important to them. You might find, after reading this book, that going into an art gallery is going to be a totally new experience for you!

3. Relate the projections to the artist

So after the viewer has made a substantial amount of comments, i.e. their own projections, I then ask the 'artist', the person who drew the picture, if they can relate to the comments – only the comments just made by the viewer.

To the reader/you – Do you relate to what your friend or family member has said about your picture, and if you do, please share with them? If you don't, that is OK too.

Note: During this process we can learn how to rid ourselves of other people's projections. I teach my clients to reject projections if it doesn't suit them and this part of the process is an opportune moment to do that. For example, if somebody in the group said that " . . . your picture looks shit, messy and makes me want to run away", instead of feeling hurt and misunderstood, you now understand, (because the viewer is projecting), that 'the viewer' feels that his life is, 'shit, messy at the moment and he wants to run away from it all', and he may well have shared this feeling in the step before (2.). Therefore, you have the freedom to say, "Sorry, but I don't relate to this at all, as my picture is, for example "about love and forgiveness." However, you might actually relate to the negative projections as well, and find that you also want to 'run away from it all'. This is something that is really hard to do in real life when you are in a group or gathering, because so much is going on. People could be talking over the top of each other and some have their own issues that they project onto you, which you don't realise at the time. But in our group art therapy process it is very obvious because we have already identified the projections of 'the viewer', so we can feel more confident in rejecting the content if it does not relate. However, you can also accept the ideas and let them enhance your life by allowing yourself to accept something that might be true. *This is one of the great advantages of groups in general. We can learn from each other, and see things we might not have noticed otherwise.*

To reinforce, what I have just said, I always ensure that the 'artist' understands that the descriptions were only projections, and the projections don't necessarily relate to them, but if they do, then they can also add a new perspective. The viewers' feedback may inspire them to think in other terms.

Now, ask yourself

Reader/you, can you see . . . (add here the words that your viewer has used before, like, for example, hope, movement, simplicity, closeness, etc.) . . . in your picture?

Does that resonate with you? Do you relate to that?

Is that what is in your life right now?

Is that what you need at the moment or would like to have more in the future?

Tell me about it.

4.   *The artist describes what is important*

It's time to leave the projections behind and have a look at what the artist sees in his or her picture. Art therapy as usual, but we need to keep it short and to the point, as we are in a large group.

We can ask the artist to describe the picture he or she has drawn, and see what other descriptions come up, beyond what the viewer has seen.

Now, your friend or partner can ask you some questions about your picture

What else do you see in your picture that is important to you? Write the answers down.

5.   *Relate the descriptions back to the artist's life*

How do the descriptions you wrote down, relate to your life in the moment? This is the main question here. "In your life, how does . . . relate to you, in the moment?"

Now, your friend or partner can ask you this question and note down your answers

6.   *The artist can choose someone else's picture*

The final step only applies to an actual group. Now, the art therapist would ask the artist to select another person's picture, not his or her own, but from the remaining group. It needs to be a picture that has not been discussed yet, so everyone gets a turn. Repeat the process from 1–5 until all pictures have been discussed.

Six-step summary of the Group Mural

1 Client A, any group member, chooses a picture from someone else in the group, client B. Then client A describes clients B's picture to the group. 2–5 minutes.
2 The art therapist asks client A how the projections relate to his/her life, client A's life.
3 The art therapist now asks client B (artist of the picture) how the described projections of client A relates back to them (*e.g. Can you, client B, relate to what you have heard from A; does this relate to your life?*).
4 Next, the art therapist asks client B to describe their own picture, not the projections of A.
5 The art therapist then asks client B how these descriptions relate to his/her life and to share some of this with the group, as long as it feels comfortable sharing. No pressure, but genuine interest.
6 Back to the start: art therapist now asks client B to choose somebody else's picture and the whole process starts again.

Some topics for the Group Mural

This technique is useful for groups because it is playful and allows for social interaction in a safe context and uncovers unconscious material in various ways. The topics that can be used are endless. Here are some examples:

- Picture frame
- Colours
- Shapes
- Senses
- Elements
- Rooms of the house
- Animals
- Trees
- Fruit

When selecting a topic consider 'what do I want to achieve for my group?' There are general topics you can use with any group (see above), but there are also topics that might be group specific, like for a new parents' group, for example, sleepless nights, relationship issues, new demands, financial issues, etc.

Group Mural: example

Gail drew a picture of what was important to her in her life and Beth, (viewer) chose the picture.

Beth: Well this picture reminds me of a holiday that I had with my family when I was growing up as a teenager. It's a very peaceful picture, very pastel and light and feels so serene and gentle. It's like many holidays I've had as a child, when it was fun to be at the beach. There's a house on the beach that is just like the house we used to stay in; it was a really nice place. But we don't go to the beach anymore.

Rob: What in your life is peaceful, serene and gentle? Is that the holiday experience or something you are experiencing now or would like more of?

Beth: It was something I experienced very strongly back then. And this picture reminds me of that time. There's a girl with a baby and a small boy and this could easily be my best friend and her baby, and my little brother. But in the centre the two figures, one of them is wearing a pale orange dress, and it kind of could be me with blonde hair, and she is kind of leaning into the person next to her, who is taller, and on her right. And that person looks like my older sister. I really like this picture a lot, because it's so serene and peaceful, but the figure in the centre who looks like my sister . . . is very disturbing.

Rob: What is disturbing about it?

Beth: Well it's my sister that is disturbing, she calls me a lot on the phone, needing my help and we go over and over her problem. She's just a mess because she was raped a long time ago and she hasn't been able to find a way to get past it. She's become an alcoholic, and I can't help her. I feel like that's me in the picture leaning into her, the one with the orange dress . . . and she's ignoring me. I want to help her but I can't. It's like this picture is the last holiday we had before things got really bad with her. I have another sister who was also very disturbed, and she committed suicide. So I'm really taken back to a time that was really peaceful and good, and serene and nice, and even innocent, and it all changed. For me, things worked out, and I've been lucky, but for my sisters, it was terrible. It really broke the family apart. But this is still a very nice, happy and lovely picture.

I then asked Gail, the artist of the picture to comment.

Rob: So tell me, do you relate to what Beth has said about your picture? Do you experience something serene, peaceful and gentle in your life, perhaps something disturbing?

Gail: Well not all of it, but I agree . . . my picture is very pastel, and pale, and soft and kind of gentle. And it is about a good time that I've had with my son, when he was a baby, and also when he was a toddler. I tried to draw what it used to be like then and what it is like now, that he is a teenager. The figures in the centre, that is me on the left leaning into him, but I am a bit disturbed by the fact that Beth thinks it's her sister, because to me, that is my son, however, he is going through some problems at the moment and we are not communicating very well, so that is very hard for me to deal with.

Rob: Do you want it to be more like it was in the past when you were at the beach?

Gail:	Yes, I do. It was easier, simpler. But now . . . I tried to show that we are well connected and close, but in the picture, I'm leaning onto him. I really don't like the way I'm leaning on him. I didn't see that before.
Rob:	What is it about leaning onto him in the picture that you don't like?
Gail:	I'm his mother. I can't lean on him. This picture is very pretty and nice and pastel, but it's also weak . . . the lines are too soft and weak.
Rob:	Do you feel weak and too soft about something?
Gail:	Yes, I hadn't realised how weak I feel about this situation with my son, who won't talk to me, and who kind of ignores what I say. I need to put space between me and my son. Draw him a bit further away. I don't want to lean on him. I realise I've got to let go, a bit more; he is a teenager. He doesn't need me to be in his face all the time asking him questions. I didn't see that before, but now looking at this picture, it really makes me see that sometimes we can't help people we love. I've got to change my attitude towards my son. I can't help him . . . with the way I am. I can't change him. I just have to be supportive, that's all. I've just been wanting things to stay the same, like when he was small and when we went to the beach, but he's growing up and I have to let go. I need to give him space to grow.

Now, it was Gail's turn to choose somebody else's picture and the Group Mural process continued from there.

Group drawing: the benefits

By our very nature we live to be part of, or connected, to other people to gain a sense of belonging, a sense of togetherness, which is fundamental to our self-esteem and survival. Our own awareness of self can often be amplified in the presence of 'others', giving us a sense of who we truly are and what potential for change lies in us. Often, people break ties with one another, with groups, with spouses and families, if they are 'unable to be loved and accepted' (Cast & Burke, 2002), or if their skills are no longer valuable, and the beliefs no longer feel right for the individual.

Working with clients or groups who are mature and respectful and responsible is quite different from working with a group who are disadvantaged, who might have been abused as children or come from broken homes, or where love and respect or guidance are minimal or non-existent. When I was first starting out as an art therapist and Pastoral Referent in a German parish, one of my jobs was working with a group of teenage boys, who were very rough, sarcastic, and negative. Most had fathers who were in jail, drug-dependent, or never there. These boys saw themselves as heading on the same path, with very little hope. Their future looked bleak, to them, and they were either very reserved in their behaviour, or loud and outspoken. I had only worked with them for a few weeks, and was making very little progress. Art for them was "sissy" and "for girls". I had put off doing the Group Mural, as I felt they weren't ready for this activity, that they might not care to listen to each other, or could possibly get into a fight. However, I really wanted this group to get better connected, as they weren't kind towards each other, and they didn't support one another at all. There was always one boy, Jake, who would be extremely disruptive and would almost always destroy the mood with put downs and aggressive behaviour.

After re-evaluating their situation, I figured we could try a very simple group drawing, where they painted one picture, together. I taped a very large piece of paper onto the wall, and laid out Caran D'Ache Neocolor I oil crayons. I asked them to draw with only one colour at a time, in abstract, and take turns and be supportive of each other. It was difficult to get them motivated, another one of their issues, and no one wanted to be first. In fact, they asked me to make the first mark. I told them it was their drawing as a group, and as 'the art therapist' I would stay out to make sure everyone is safe. "You can do anything", I said, hoping this affected them in a positive way. Finally, one of the more creative and quiet boys got up, and took a crayon and the noise in the room died down. Everyone watched intently, and after he had finished drawing which only took a couple of minutes, the others were now inspired to get up after him and draw as well. Some made quick, rough marks and others spent a bit of time with it. But it was fascinating for them to watch each other doing the drawing, to see it evolve. At times I had to encourage them to come up and draw, but all of them joined in, made positive comments about each other's marks, and their usual sarcasm and negativity was quite minimal.

Jake, had been up a few times already, but was probably not getting as much attention as he normally does by being disruptive, and it was his turn again. He got up, went over to the drawing, picked up a black crayon and started working into it very roughly, saying, "I don't like this, I don't like it at all", going over and over the whole drawing and covering everything in a very dark colour. A few of the others were getting upset about what he was doing to their drawing, telling him to stop. The more they protested the more Jake worked into it with the black colour. Jake then looked at what he had done, didn't like it and ripped the paper off the wall, scrunched it up and threw it on the floor. I wanted to intercept but stopped myself. The boys collectively sorted the situation out themselves, like I'd never seen before. One of them picked up the paper and reprimanded Jake for his aggressive behaviour. They put the drawing back up on the wall, and then decided to change it, "Fix it", so that they had a, "A better picture". Each one of them took turns to go up again and add more to the drawing, and with each turn, the comments were supportive, "That looks better", and "I know, let's do this", and "I think we can fix it". There was a greater feeling of support, and a cohesion in the group that wasn't there at the start of the session. Even though Jake had upset them with his negativity, they, for once, wouldn't allow it. Their own individual desire to create something, a work of art, had inspired them to collectively honour and support each other in the group. They showed courage in standing up to Jake, something they normally didn't do. Jake later commented to the group about how he felt, and said he realised that he, "didn't want to wreck the drawing", but he couldn't stop the "bad feelings". This is something that often happens to him in groups. I met with this group of boys over the next few months, and even though they were still back to their old ways at times, their sense of belonging and their sense of self was starting to change. We managed to continue our group art therapy, often using Group Murals, which gave them many insights along the way, and a new direction that started to transform their lives.

Final thoughts

I hope this book has been a good companion, and that you can refer to it often, and utilise the ideas to suit your needs. My intention was to give you the best practical ideas of how to work with clients in individual and group contexts, as well as giving you insights into yourself, through art therapy. Even though life often sets us new challenges and some difficult problems and situations, taking care of yourself and your clients is an ongoing process, a journey beyond words and back to words, where you can become more conscious of some of your unconscious content. Scary or not, most likely liberating, and more mindful of your potential. I hope you find that the step-by-step art therapy techniques and ideas help you along the way, and transform your world into a better place, unleashing a more positive approach towards life for you and your clients.

May your journey continue creatively and with inspiration,

Rob G.

Literature

Case, C., & Dalley, T. (2014). *The handbook of art therapy* (3rd ed.). London, New York: Routledge, Taylor & Francis Group.

Cast, A.D. & Burke, P.J. (2002). A theory of self-esteem. *Social Forces 80*(3), 1041–1068.

Liebmann, M. (2004). *Art therapy for groups* (2nd ed.). London, New York: Brunner, Routledge.

Malchiodi, C. (2007). *The art therapy sourcebook*. New York. McGraw-Hill.

Malchiodi, C.A. (2012). *Handbook of art therapy* (2nd ed.). London, New York: The Guildford Press.

McNeilly, G. (2005). *Group analytic art therapy*. London, Philadelphia: Jessica Kingsley.

Skaife, S. & Huet, V. (1998). *Art psychotherpay groups*. London: Routledge.

Spreti, F. v., Martius, P. & Foerstl, H. (2012). *Art therapy with psychological disorders* (trans.) (2nd ed.). Munich: Urban & Fischer.

Ulman, E. (2016). Variations on a Freudian theme. In J.A. Rubin (Ed.), *Approaches to art therapy: Theory and technique* (pp. 106–125) (3rd ed.). New York, Oxon: Routledge.

Waller, D. (2014). *Group interactive art therapy: Its use in training and treatment*. London, New York: Routledge.

Wilson, L. & Betensky, M. (2016). Art is the therapy. In J.A. Rubin (Ed.), *Approaches to art therapy: Theory and technique* (pp. 17–32) (3rd ed.). New York, Oxon: Routledge.

Pseudonyms

There are many examples in this book of different approaches that were used with clients or students. To protect their privacy, I have changed their names and sometimes small details of their stories.

Acknowledgments

I am very grateful to the many lecturers, supervisors and students who have helped me to achieve this book, and to all those remarkable art therapists worldwide who have put their ideas into words for publication. I owe a lot to my art therapy lecturers, mentors and supervisors, as much of my work is developed from their approaches and ideas. Foremost, I would like to acknowledge Brigitte Held, Ludwig Seyfried, Otto Hanus and Flora von Spreti who have been extremely creative in their use and development of art therapy and whose knowledge has been invaluable. Many of the techniques I discussed in this book are profoundly influenced by them. I would also like to express my gratitude to Francine Hoitink for her feedback, and Joan Garvan for proofreading and always knowing where to put the commas. A very special thanks goes to Vee Malnar for editing and taking on whatever I threw her way, for her amazing creative input, thinking like a true art therapist and making sense of what my German and complex mind was really trying to say.

Last, but not least, the biggest thanks goes to my wife, Katrina, who has put up with me being in my office far too long. I've been wading through books, behind a computer screen and sticking my head through the door at times, like our guinea pigs when it is feeding time. Her love, support and encouragement is, in the end, what made this book possible.

Index

References to illustrations are indicated in *italics*.

abstract art and self-picture mind map:
  Abstract Art 67; abstract art and therapy
  67–68; abstract self-picture drawing
  task 68–69; describe your self-picture
  69; explore colours 71–72, 78; explore
  forms, shapes and lines 70; explore light
  74; explore movement and lines 72–73;
  explore space and relationship 73–74;
  explore texture and sensual aspects
  74–75; mind mapping of descriptions or
  themes 75–76, *75*; order your mind map
  76–77; relating story to client's life/current
  issues 77; self-picture of Melissa 78
acceptance and commitment therapy
  (ACT) 114
analytical psychology 1, 48
anxiety disorders, and Life Scripts 52–53
Aristotle 48
Amhem Land rock markings 1
'art as therapy' model: beginnings (1930s)
  10, 11; characteristics of approach 2–3,
  4, 12; comparison with 'art in therapy'
  11–12; and group therapy 128; and
  Inner Resources technique 19–20

art education, and psycho education 72
'art in therapy' (art psychotherapy)
  model: beginnings (1940s) 10, 11;
  characteristics of approach 2–3, 4,
  12–13; comparison with 'art as therapy'
  model 11–12; and group therapy 128;
  and House-Tree-Person (HTP) task
  32–33; and Inner Resources technique
  20–22; need for detail in images 57; and
  self-picture mind map with abstract art
  68, 69–70, 71–72, 77
art psychotherapy *see* 'art in therapy' (art
  psychotherapy) model
art therapy: beginnings 10, 11; and
  cognitive behaviour therapy (CBT) 3–4,
  8, 9; as key to unlocking unconscious
  1; and neuroscience 93–94; origin of
  term 11; psychology and art therapy
  official timeline 10; and transference/
  countertransference work 13–14; *see also*
  'art as therapy' model; 'art in therapy'
  (art psychotherapy) model; art therapy
  and cognitive behaviour therapy (CBT);
  group art therapy; positive art therapy

art therapy and cognitive behaviour therapy (CBT): arguments for art therapy in conjunction with CBT 112–114; art therapy and CBT throughout this book 125; guidance for psychologists, art therapists and readers 114; sequence 1: unwanted cognition: instructions and Ana's example 114–117, *115*; sequence 2: doubt: instructions and Ana's example 117–120, *120*; sequence 3: fusion of unwanted cognition with doubt: instructions and Ana's example 120–121, *121*; sequence 4: wanted cognition: instructions and Ana's example 121–122, *122*; sequence 5: positive consequences: instructions and Ana's example 123–124, *123*; sequence 6: fusion of wanted cognition and positive consequences: instructions and Ana's example 124, *124*; sequence 7: review 124–125; sequence 8: possible additional work 125; *see also* cognitive behaviour therapy (CBT)

Asmundson, G. 113
attachment disorders 52
'awarefulness' *see* mindfulness ('awarefulness')

Bandura, Albert 9
Beck, Aaron 9
behavioural therapy 9, 10; *see also* art therapy and cognitive behaviour therapy (CBT); cognitive behaviour therapy (CBT); dialectical behavioural therapy (DBT)
Berne, Eric 43, 44
Betensky, M. 69
Bowlby, J. 52
brain: and art-related experiences 93–94; 'flight or fight' inbuilt response 20; left-brain/right-brain thinking 9; neurological pathways 94–95, 104–105, 106, 107–109; 'second brain' concept 13; traumatic brain injury (TBI) 94; and traumatic experiences 80, 86
Breuer, Josef 30
Bridle, Dean 93

Buck, John N. 30, 33, 36–37
Buddha 84

Case, Caroline 9, 11, 127, 129
cave paintings 1, 11
CBT *see* art therapy and cognitive behaviour therapy (CBT); cognitive behaviour therapy (CBT)
Cézanne, Paul 67
change, and personal growth 84
clay work 26
client-centred therapy (C. Rogers) 11, 24, 52, 74
Code of Conduct 110
cognitive behaviour therapy (CBT): and art therapy 3–4, 8, 9; and art therapy throughout this book 125; beginnings (1970s) 10; and Inner Resources technique 22; and psychoanalysis, differences and similarities 9–10; and S.M.A.R.T. goal-setting strategy 56–57, 59, 64; and unconscious 7–8; *see also* art therapy and cognitive behaviour therapy (CBT)
cognitive empathy 24
cognitive therapy 9, 10; *see also* art therapy and cognitive behaviour therapy (CBT); cognitive behaviour therapy (CBT); mindfulness-based cognitive therapies (MBCT)
collective unconscious 60–61
colours, and emotions 71–72, 78
Comer, R.J. 113
Confucius 48
countertransference 10, 11, 13–14, 24, 33
Creative Mind Ordering (CMO): art therapy and neuroscience 93–94; changing neural pathways 94–95, 104–105, 106, 107–109; diagram of CMO process *109*; step 1: trigger, drawing and descriptions 95–98, *97*; step 2: symptom, drawing and descriptions 95, 98–102, *100*; step 3: inner strength, drawing and descriptions 95, 102–104, *103*; step 4: fusion, drawing and descriptions 95, 104–106, *105*; step 5: decision, drawing and descriptions 95, 106–108, *108*; Tania example (step 1) 97–98, *97*;

Tania example (step 2) 99–102, *100*;
Tania example (step 3) 103–104, *103*;
Tania example (step 4) *105*, 106; Tania
example (step 5) 108, *108*; when and
when not using CMO 110
Csikszentmihalyi, Mihaly 18, 20
Cubism 67
Curtis, E.K. 69

Dali, Salvador 14
Dalley, Tessa 9, 11, 127, 129
depression: and goal-directed activities 65;
and Inner Resources technique 23–24;
and repressed emotions 8
dialectical behavioural therapy (DBT) 114
dishonest compliances 37
dreams, as access code to unconscious 1–2

early childhood Inner Resources *see* Inner
Resources Technique
Ellis, Albert 9, 114
emotions: and colours 71–72, 78; and
Life Scripts technique 53; and the
unconscious 8
empathy, cognitive empathy 24
epigenetics 61

feeling picture cards 72; *see also* emotions
'flight or fight' inbuilt response 20
foundations: emotions and the
unconscious 8; Freud's understanding
of the unconscious 7–8, 10; interpreting
14–15; psychoanalysis and cognitive
behaviour therapy compared 9–10;
psychology and art therapy official
timeline 10; two types of art therapy
11–14; using this book 6
free association 12–13, 14, 21, 53, 57
Freud, Sigmund: dreams as access
code to unconscious 1; dreams
experienced in visual images 2;
free association 14, 21; id/
superego/ego theory 43; imagery
as means to make unconscious
conscious 8; psychosexual stages of
development 36; and Surrealism 67;
talking cure 30; unconscious, theory
of 7–8, 10; views of influenced by
European philosophy 9

George, Saint 87
Gestalt therapy 80, 81
goals: cognitive behaviour therapy and
S.M.A.R.T. strategy 56–57, 59, 64;
Goal Drawing exercise 57–58, 61,
63, 65; Jennifer's Goal *58*, 59, 60,
61–62, 63, 64; looking for evidence
in drawing 59–60; obstacles and
collective unconscious 60–62;
strengths 62–63; therapeutic process
65; use of therapy with depressed and
young clients 65–66
group art therapy: different approaches
and groups 127–128; *see also* Group
Mural Technique
Group Mural Technique: concept
128, *128*; drawing instructions 129;
example of group drawing (Jake and
group of boys) 135–137; example
of Group Mural discussion (Gail
and Beth) 133–135; group rules and
confidentiality 129; picture composition
to form mural 129; six-step process
129–132; six-step process summary
133; topics and selection of 133
gut feeling (of therapist) 13, 53, 76

Hanus, Otto 69–70, 95, 114
happiness 17–18
Hawker, S. 8
'health and art' groups 2
Held, Brigitte 18, 45
Heraclitus 84
Herman, J.L. 80
Hill, Adrian 1, 11
Hofmann, S. 113
House-Tree-Person (HTP) task: Buck's H-T-P
theory 30, 33, 36–37; case of John 34;
case of Natalie 38–42, *38*; case of Sarah
35–36; case of Steve 34–35; drawing
31–32; duration of task 31; limitations
and precautions 37–38; questions to ask
about drawing 32–33; studies on HTP
methods 30–31; theoretical origins of HTP
36; typical issues and populations 36–37;
visualisation 31
Huet, V. 127
humanistic therapy 10; *see also* client-
centred therapy (C. Rogers)

Huna Principle (energy flows where attention goes) 87, 107
Hurricane Katrina, and trauma work with children 84
Huss, E. 112

imagery: as alternative medium for expression 2; and dreams 1–2; figurative vs abstract images 37; as means to make unconscious conscious 8; psychological effects of 1; representational images 31, 36, 52
inner adult principle 43–44
inner child principle 43–44
Inner Resources Technique: case of Daniel 26–27; case of Emma 24–26, *24*; clay work 26; depressed clients 23–24; duration of task and materials 18–19; further work 26; instructions 19; "It's a good feeling" exercise 20–21, 22; look for the positive 20; process 19; reflections 19–20; senses and link to *now* 21–22; themes and questions 20; therapy 22; trauma work 23
inner scripts 44
inner wise man/woman principle 44
interpreting 14–15, 21
interpsychic conflicts 43–44

Jung, Carl Gustav: collective unconscious 60–61; dreams as access code to unconscious 1; extreme positions vs balance 48; free association 21; imagery as means to make unconscious conscious 8; 'persona' concept 81; self as centre 68, 69; 'shadow' concept 87; and Surrealism 67; therapeutic process as alchemy 87; unconscious, theory of 10; *see also* Self-Box technique

Kandinsky, Wassily 67
Kinetic House-Tree-Person method (K-HTP) 30
Kinglake, Alexander William 43
Kramer, Edith 7, 11

Lascaux caves 1
left-brain thinking 9
Liebmann, M. 127

Life Scripts: Berne and interpsychic conflicts 43–44; case of anxious clients 52–53; case of Jessica 49–50, *49*; case of John 51; case of Mia 50; case of Rebecca 51; case of Sarah 51; defining inner/life script 44–45; early childhood drawing task 45; exploring the drawings (themes, rules, outcomes) 46–47; Life Script from analysis of drawings 47–48; repeating exercise for adolescence, adulthood and overall Life Scripts 54–55; reversing the Life Script 48–49; seeking feedback from clients 51–52; therapist's role 53–54

McNeilly, G. 127
McWilliams, N. 9
'making space' 6
Malchiodi, Cathy 11, 84
Management of Mental Disorders Manual 113
Marx, Karl 67
Meichenbaum, Donald 9
mind mapping *see* abstract art and self-picture mind map
mindfulness ('awarefulness') 6, 19, 57, 69, 137
mindfulness-based cognitive therapies (MBCT) 112, 113–114
Morris, J. 112
motivational interviewing (MI) 114

Naphausen, Birgit 69–70
Naumburg, Margaret 7, 11, 81
neural plasticity theory 94–95, 104–105, 106, 107–109
neurogenesis 94
neuroscience: and art therapy 93–94; neural plasticity theory 94–95, 104–105, 106, 107–109; *see also* brain
Norcross, J.C. 13

Oaklander, Violet 80
obsessive compulsive disorder (OCD), and Life Scripts 52–53

Park, N. 18
Peavy, V. 69
Perls, Fritz 81

'persona' concept 81
personality theories 36
Peterson, Ch. 18
Picasso, Pablo 78
Pollock, Jackson 78
positive art therapy: happiness and
    positive psychology 17–18; Inner
    Resources Technique 18–27; Role
    Models Technique 27–29; *see also* Inner
    Resources Technique; Role Models
    Technique
positive psychology 18
post-traumatic stress disorder
    (PTSD) 23
Prochaska, J.O. 13
projections: and Group Mural Technique
    130–133; and Role Models Technique
    27–29; of therapist 21, 33, 91;
    unconscious projections and art therapy
    vs CBT 113; unconscious projections
    and Goal Drawing exercise 57–58
projective drawings 30, 31
projectives 36
psycho education, and art education 72
psychoanalysis: beginnings (early 1900s)
    10; and cognitive behaviour therapy,
    differences and similarities 9–10; loss
    of popularity after World War II 10;
    see also Freud, Sigmund; Jung, Carl
    Gustav
psychology: psychology and art therapy
    official timeline 10; as science vs.
    psychotherapy as art 112
psychoneuroimmunology 94
psychotherapy, as art vs. psychology as
    science 112

Quail, J. 69

rational-emotive therapy (RET) 112
religions 17
representational images 31, 36, 52
resistance 9, 65, 98
right-brain thinking 9
Rogers, Carl R. 11, 24, 52, 74
Role Models Technique: defining
    projections 27–28; duration of
    task, materials and instructions 28;
    exploration of role models 28–29

rosebush strategy 80
Rubin, Judith A. 1

'second brain' concept 13
Self-Box technique: defining trauma
    and rosebush therapy 80; Jungian
    box/Self-Box theory 81; making the
    Self-Box 81–82; questions for personal
    reflections 83–84; Self-Box as process
    84; story of St George and the dragon
    87; therapeutic goal 1: become more
    authentic and example of Steph 84–85,
    88–89, *88*; therapeutic goal 2: integrate
    traumatic memories and example of
    Helena 85–87, 89–91, *89, 90*
self-picture mind map *see* abstract art and
    self-picture mind map
Seligman, M.E.P. 18
senses, and Inner Resources technique
    21–23
September 11 attacks, and trauma work 11
sexual abuse case 40–41
Seyfried, Ludwig 18, 45
'shadow' concept 87
Siegel, D.J. 21, 76, 86, 107
Skaife, S. 127
Skinner, B.F. 9
S.M.A.R.T. goal-setting strategy 56–57,
    59, 64
Socrates 17
solution-focused therapy 123
Spreti, Flora von 24, 52
Surrealism 67
Synthetic House-Tree-Person method
    (S-HTP) 30

Thomaser, Maria 69–70
Torem, M.S. 30–31
transactional analysis 43
transference 9, 10, 11, 13–14, 33; *see also*
    countertransference
trauma work: and Hurricane Katrina 84;
    and Inner Resources Technique 23; and
    September 11 attacks 11; *see also* Self-
    Box technique
traumatic brain injury (TBI) 94

unconscious: art therapy as key to
    unlocking of 1; and cognitive behaviour

therapy 7–8; collective unconscious
60–61; dreams/images as access code
to 1–2; and emotions 8; and free
association 12–13; Freud's theory 7–8,
10; Jung's theory 10; as our friend 62

Van Gogh, Vincent 18, 71, 78

Wadeson, H. 3
Waite, M. 8
Waller, D. 127
Watson, John B. 9
Wolpe, Joseph 9

Young, Jeffrey 44

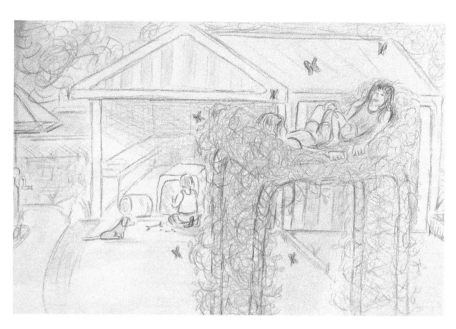

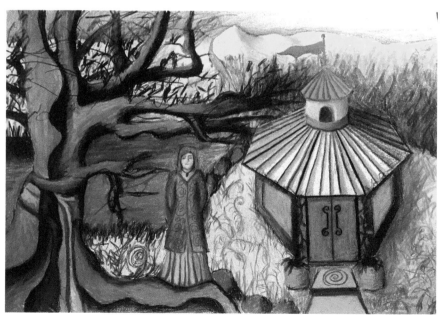

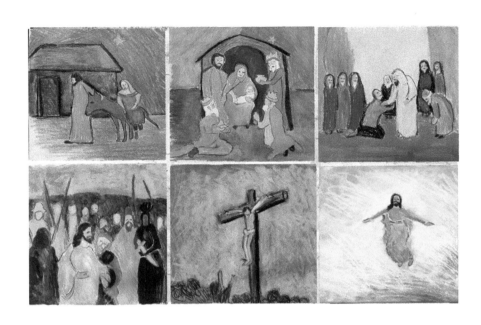

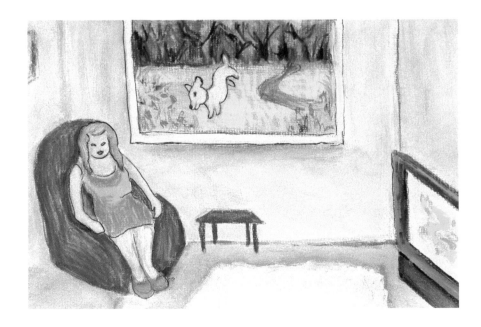

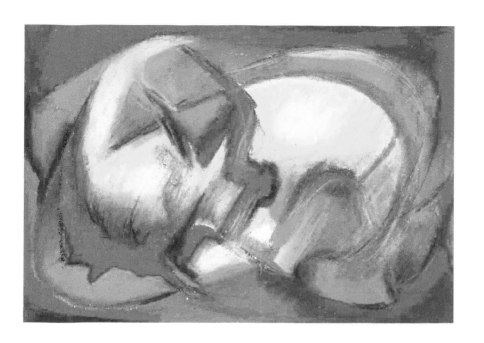

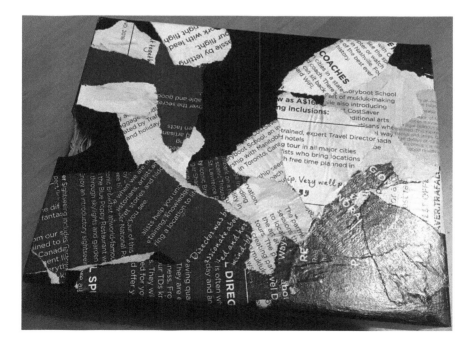

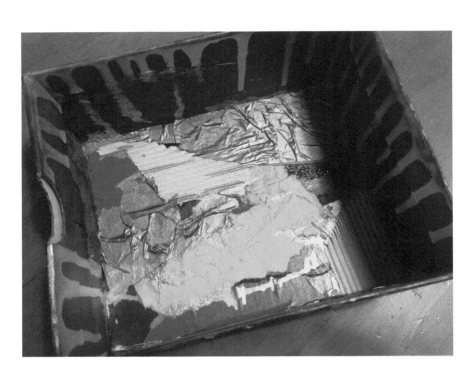

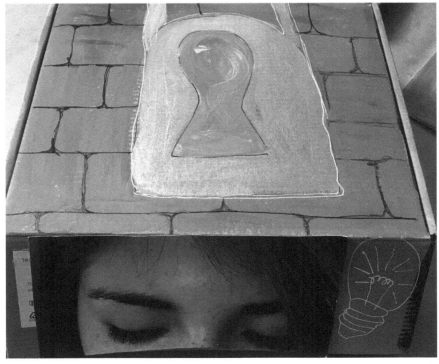

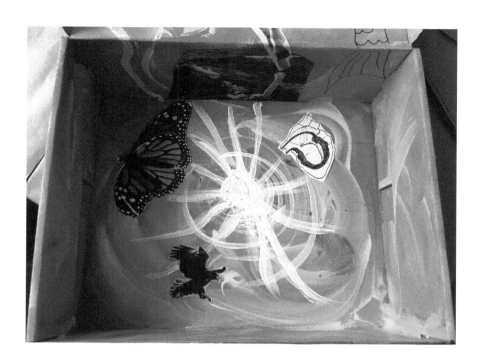

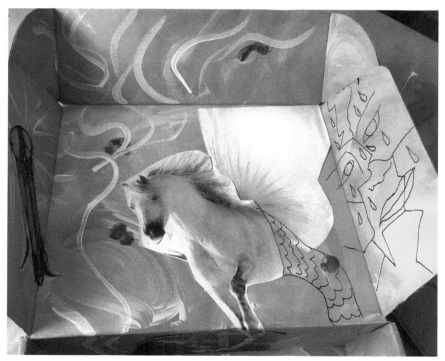

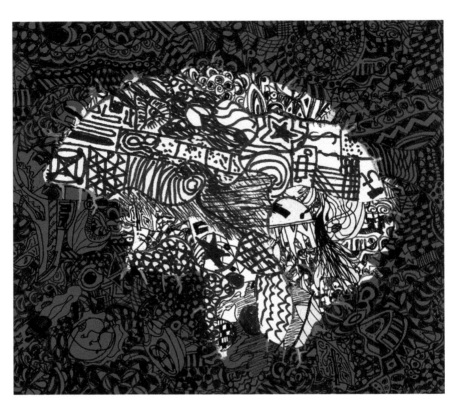

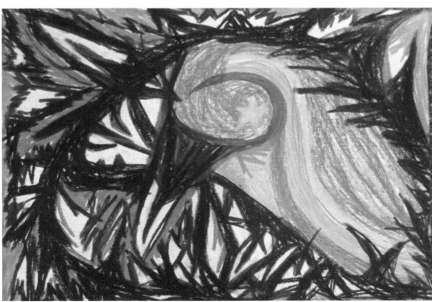

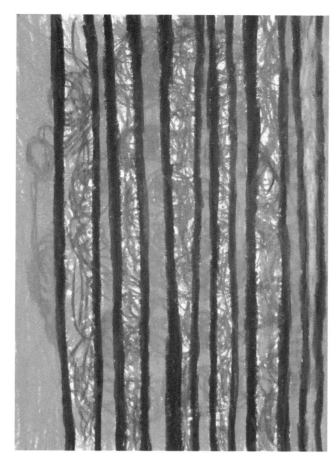

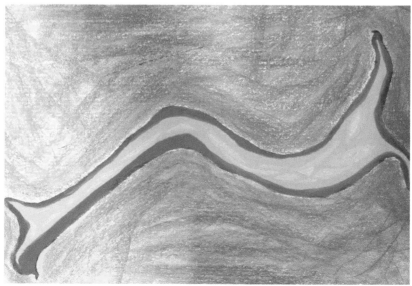

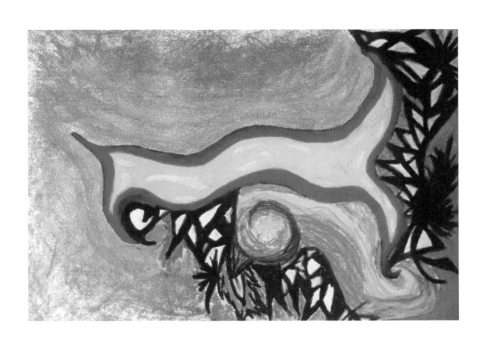

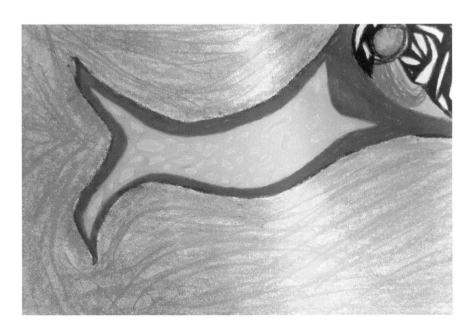

Diagram of the CMO process

* Start at the bottom with Session 1 and follow the arrows to Session 2 etc.

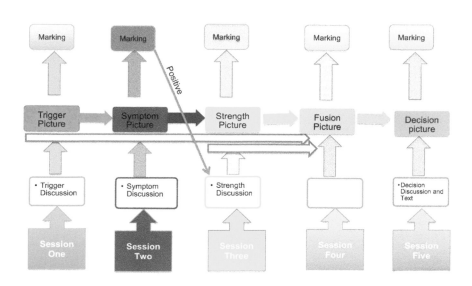

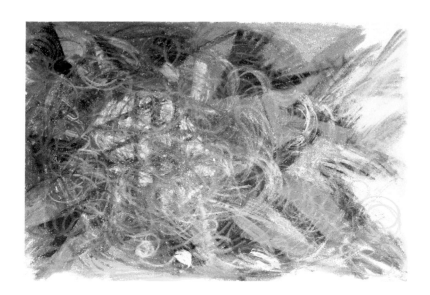

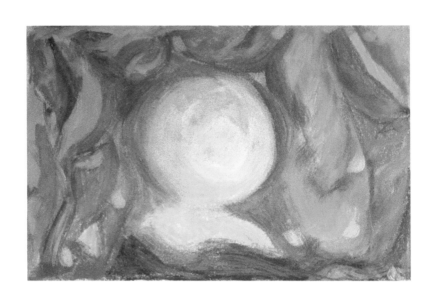

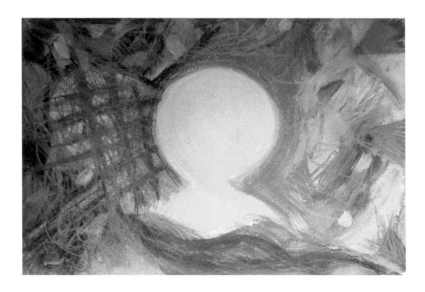

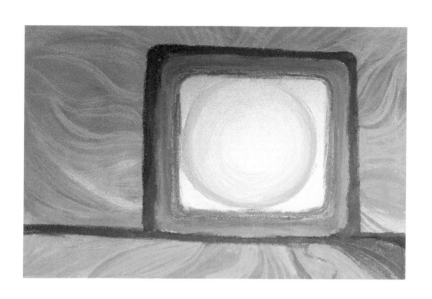

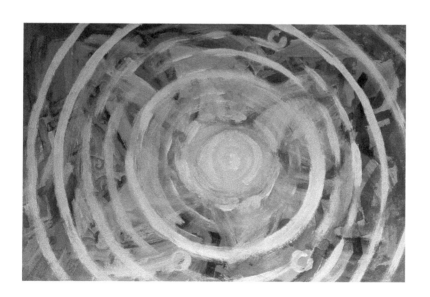

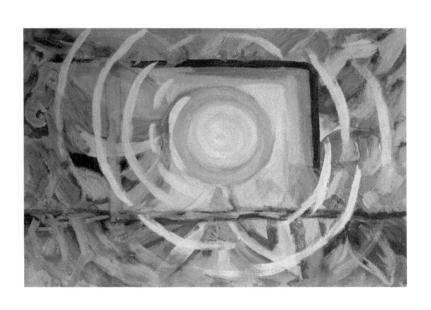

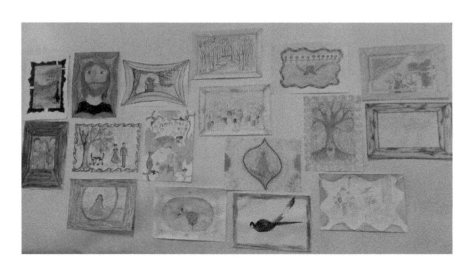

For Product Safety Concerns and Information please contact our EU
representative GPSR@taylorandfrancis.com
Taylor & Francis Verlag GmbH, Kaufingerstraße 24, 80331 München, Germany